The Nurse's Internet Handbook

a guide for nurses in primary care

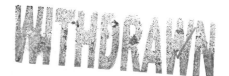

Robert Kiley

Head of Systems Strategy at the Wellcome Library for the History and
Understanding of Medicine

Elizabeth Graham

Reader Services Manager at the Wellcome Library for the History and
Understanding of Medicine

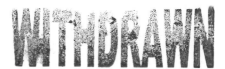

Supported by an educational grant from Sanofi Pasteur MSD

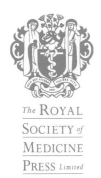

The ROYAL
SOCIETY of
MEDICINE
PRESS Limited

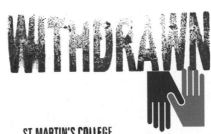

ST MARTIN'S COLLEGE
CARLISLE LIBRARY

Royal College
of Nursing
Travel Health Forum

The publisher has used its best endeavours to ensure that the URLs for the external websites referred to in this book are correct and active at the time of going to press. However, the publisher has no responsibility for the websites and can make no guarantee that a site will remain live or that the content is or will remain appropriate.

British Library Cataloguing in Publication Data
A catalogue record for this book is available from the British Library.

ISBN 1–85315–655–8

Distribution in Europe and Rest of World:
Marston Book Services Ltd
PO Box 269
Abingdon
OXON OX14 4YN, UK
Tel: +44 (0)1235 465 500
Fax: +44 (0)1235 465 555
Email: direct.order@marston.co.uk

Distribution in the USA and Canada:
Royal Society of Medicine Press Ltd
c/o Jamco Distribution Inc
1401 Lakeway Drive
Lewisville, TX 75057, USA
Tel: +1 800 538 1287
Fax: +1 972 353 1303
Email: jamco@majors.com

Distribution in Australia and New Zealand:
Elsevier Australia
30–52 Smidmore Street
Marrickville NSW 2204
Australia
Tel: + 61 2 9517 8999
Fax: + 61 2 9517 2249
Email: service@elsevier.com.au

Designed and typeset by Phoenix Photosetting, Chatham, Kent
Printed in the Netherlands by Alfabase, Alphen aan den Rijn

Contents

Foreword

The revolution in information technology has had a major impact on all our lives. For example, just 10 years ago how many of us working in the field of travel medicine would have anticipated the increased use of the Internet as we know it today? The Internet has enhanced the way people are able to learn about other countries in an exciting and interactive format; it has enabled businesses and organisations to advertise their travel experience opportunities, and many people now book their trips 'online'. In the context of a travel health consultation, this exciting medium enables us to give the latest up-to-date advice, essential in a field of medicine that is forever changing – we are now able to access government sources for guidelines and review evidence-based information to help us give the best possible advice. Travel health information databases on the Internet are invaluable in helping us and our travellers to access such information with great ease, and they enable the public to be more involved, taking greater responsibility for their own travel-related healthcare and safety.

As part of our professional code of conduct, we have a responsibility to keep ourselves up-to-date and there is no better way than using well-recognised and official websites. Indeed such information may, in the future, have limited availability in paper format so it is essential that we all become confident and able when using the Internet.

The authors of this book, Robert Kiley and Elizabeth Graham, are highly experienced in guiding readers through the principles of the Internet. Whether you are new to the concept of this technology, or someone who would like to understand the more complex applications for your professional or personal development, the content of this publication has something for you and cannot be recommended highly enough.

Jane Chiodini MSc RGN RM
Chair, RCN Travel Health Forum

Preface

A recent study[1] found that Internet use among nurses at work was low compared with other groups, despite adequate workplace access. Although the reasons cited for this were many – including the fact that nurses are more likely to value interpersonal contact, and prefer to use personal experience and communication with colleagues and patients rather than online sources – it was also recognised that lack of experience, coupled with the need to be able to find relevant information quickly, were also significant barriers to Internet use.

This handbook attempts to remove these barriers by providing a jargon-free guide to nursing information on the Internet. Specifically, we explain how to use the key Internet tools (the Web browser and email) and demonstrate how the Internet can be searched to find relevant, high-quality information in a timely fashion.

Recognising that busy health professionals do not have the time to 'surf the Web' in a serendipitous way, we also highlight a number of useful Web resources relating to topics of particular relevance to nurses in primary care. Topics covered include the 10 key disease areas of the General Medical Services (GMS) Contract as well as specific chapters on childhood immunisation and travel health. The book also includes a practical guide on how you can use the Internet to find peer-reviewed research, using online bibliographic databases, such as Medline and CINAHL. The final chapter looks at the quality of health information on the Internet and, more importantly, explains how you can develop critical appraisal skills to help sort the good sites from the bad.

Inevitably, this book contains many Web addresses – URL's. To provide easy access to these sites and to save you the bother of having to key-in these addresses all the resources mentioned here can be reached through the specially created Web site: <http://www.nurseshandbook.co.uk>.

The Internet contains a wealth of information of interest and relevance to nurses in primary care. Using the tools, techniques and sites discussed in this text we hope that the time you spend on the Internet will be fruitful, efficient and enjoyable.

Robert Kiley & Elizabeth Graham
2005

---

1. Eastabrooks CA, O'Leary KA, Ricker KL, Humphrey CK. The Internet and access to evidence: how are nurses positioned? *Journal of Advanced Nursing* 2003; **42**: 73. Freely available on the Internet at: <http://www.blackwell-synergy.com/links/doi/10.1046/j.1365-2648.2003.02581.x/enhancedabs/>

About the authors

Robert Kiley is Head of Systems Strategy at the Wellcome Library for the History and Understanding of Medicine. He has written a number of related books including 'Medical information on the Internet: a guide for health professionals' (Churchill Livingstone, 3rd edn. 2003) and the 'Doctor's Internet Handbook' (RSM Press, 2000). He also edited the bi-monthly journal 'He@lth Information on the Internet' from 1998 to 2000.

Kiley is a frequent commentator on health/internet issues and has appeared on BBC World and BBC Radio 4.

Elizabeth Graham is Reader Services Manager at the Wellcome Library for the History and Understanding of Medicine. With Kiley she co-authored the 'Patient's Internet Handbook' (RSM Press, 2002). She is an experienced Internet user and has run a number of training courses on how to search the Internet effectively.

The Internet: an introduction

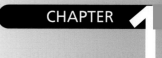

CHAPTER 1

Box 1.1   Chapter objectives

♦ Outline the structure of the book.

♦ Provide a no-nonsense, jargon-free introduction to the Internet.

♦ Discuss the types of information and services available on the Internet.

♦ Highlight the wealth of resources available to nurses working in primary care.

Introduction

Unless you have been living on another planet these past few years, it cannot have escaped your notice that the whole world appears to be obsessed by the Internet. Even when you are nowhere near a computer you cannot completely hide from this new medium. Radio presenters implore you to 'listen again' to your favourite programmes via the Web, whilst virtually every TV programme ends with an invitation to visit the show's Web site where further information etc. can be found. Even if you avoid all this, every shop you visit, or service you use, encourages you to visit their Web site. And, in a development never envisaged when the Internet was developed, hostage-takers are now using this medium to broadcast their demands and, more gruesomely, videos of what happens to their victims when these are not met.

In terms of health information, the Internet has had a massive impact on both health professionals and consumers. Anyone with an Internet connection can, at the touch of a button, access the latest research papers, clinical trials data, drug information and a whole host of patient advocacy sites, ranging from good, high-quality sources, through to sites that contain information that is both inaccurate and dangerous.

Indeed, it is the sheer volume of information, of varying quality, which may stop many users – including primary care nurses – from using the Internet. A simple Internet search for, say, diabetes, identifies over 13 million Web pages. If this was not bad enough, the searcher also has to come to grips with Internet tools – a Web browser, email software etc. – and, as previously alluded to, learn how to sort the wheat from the chaff. Faced with these challenges it is not surprising that many busy healthcare professionals decide that they can live without the Internet.

The Internet, however, contains much information that is of interest to primary care nurses. It is the purpose of this book, therefore, to demonstrate this, and encourage you to make use of this new and dynamic information source. We intend to do this by:

◆ providing a simple, jargon-free guide to the Internet
◆ explaining how to use the key Internet tools – the Web browser and email
◆ demonstrating, through relevant examples, how the Internet can be searched to find relevant, high-quality information in a timely fashion
◆ highlighting a number of resources relating to topics of particular relevance to nurses in primary care.

Using this book

To provide a clear navigational structure to the book we have divided the contents into three discrete sections. This allows you to dip into those sections that you find most relevant.

Section 1 – Introduction to the Internet: a beginners guide

This section provides an introduction to the Internet, a guide to using a Web browser and sending and receiving email, and an overview of Web searching. Although these chapters will appeal to new users, by the inclusion of topics such as managing junk mail (spam) and computer viruses, it is hoped that the more experienced user will also find information that is of use.

Section 2 – The Nursing Web

This section introduces you to a selection of high-quality resources relating to topics of particular relevance to nurses in primary care. Topics covered include the 10 key disease areas of the General Medical Services (GMS) Contract as well as specific chapters on childhood immunisation and travel health.

Section 3 – The Internet for primary care nurses – advanced skills

This final section looks at how you can use the Internet to undertake more research-based searches using databases such as Medline, and CINAHL.

The section concludes with an analysis of the quality of health information on the Internet and, more importantly, explains how you can develop critical appraisal skills to help sort the good sites from the bad and downright ugly.

About the book

Throughout the book we will avoid, wherever possible, the use of jargon. When there is no alternative the term will be highlighted – indicating that an explanation of this concept is provided in the glossary.

Each chapter will be prefaced by a set of objectives. These will help you to decide whether or not a chapter is relevant to your interests or needs. To help you get a feel for the Internet, the book also includes a number of screen shots. These are particularly useful when discussing topics such as how to search the Internet or send email, as they provide a visual, step-by-step guide, which you can follow and repeat on your own computer. A number of 'Top Tips' will also be provided. These will be shown as follows:

> *Although addresses are shown as http://www.whatever.com – you can leave out the http:// when entering the address into your web browser.*

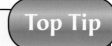

Top Tip

Inevitably a book about the Internet will contain a number of Internet addresses – URL's as they are known. To provide easy access to the sites discussed in this book – and to save you the bother of having to key-in these addresses – all the resources mentioned here can be reached through the following Web site: <http://www.nurseshandbook.co.uk>.

Already though we are getting ahead of ourselves. Before we start exploring the Internet, let us take a step back and look at what the Internet is, and what type of information and services it provides access to.

What is the Internet?

The Internet is just a system of computer networks that spans the globe. What makes the Internet so remarkable is the fact that all these computers, on all these separate networks, can all communicate with each other.

For the beginner, perhaps the most important concept to grasp is there is no central 'Internet computer'. For example, when you require a document published by the National Institutes of Health you obtain it directly (via the Internet and your Web browser) from a computer (known as a server) located within the NIH. Similarly, to see this week's edition of the British Medical Journal (*BMJ*) produced by the BMA, you access a computer run by the BMA.

What can I access through the Internet?

Box 1.2 provides an example of the range of services and information sources available via the Internet. This is, however, just a sample of what you can do via the Internet. Indeed, almost anything you might want to know

Box 1.2 Sample of information sources and services available via the Internet

♦ Online banking. Pay bills and manage your finances from your desktop (Figure 1.1).
♦ Shopping. Let Tescos <http://www.tesco.com> come to you.
♦ Holidays. Find a last minute bargain <http://www.lastminute.com>.
♦ News. Keep up-to-date with the latest news from around the world <http://news.bbc.co.uk> (Figure 1.2).
♦ Films. Preview the latest films <http://www.odeon.co.uk/>

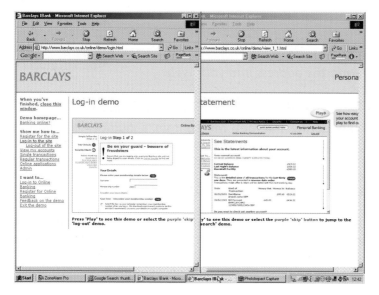

Figure 1.1 *Online banking – from Barclays*

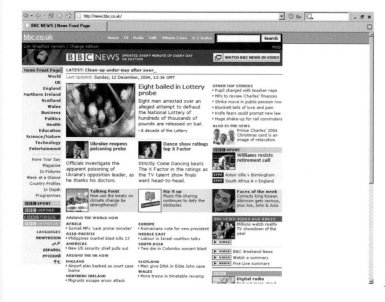

Figure 1.2 *The latest world news from the BBC*

can be found on the Internet, whilst virtually every kind of service– from shopping, through to completing your tax return and renewing your library books – can be conducted through the Internet.

Recognising the benefits of e-government, (such as greater choice, convenience, speed, and accessibility), the UK government has set a target that 100% of its services should be available online by 31 December 2005. Although this date will probably slip, it will not be too long before we can book appointments with our GP's or access local planning applications via the Internet.

The Internet for primary care nurses

In addition to the raft of general services that are available, the Internet also provides access to a wealth of information sources that can help you keep up-to-date with your professional interests.

Perhaps the best way to demonstrate the power and potential of the Internet is through an example. **Box 1.3** highlights some of the resources that can be found in response to a query about childhood immunisation.

This single example not only demonstrates the range of materials that is available on the Internet, it also serves to show how established information sources – such as journals and patient information leaflets – have migrated to this new medium, where they have been joined by numerous other resources (eg videos) that before the development of the Internet would have been unavailable.

Box 1.3   Childhood immunisation: some relevant Internet resources

♦ Information for parents, from the NHS Immunisation Information, about childhood immunisation <http://www.immunisation.nhs.uk/>

♦ Vaccine administration data from the Vaccine Information Service <http://www.spmsd.co.uk/vis_online/>

♦ Citations and abstracts relating to childhood immunisation from the PubMED MEDLINE database <http://www.pubmed.gov>.

♦ A full-text article from the evidence-based medicine journal, *Bandolier*, on the benefits and risks of MMR <http://www.jr2.ox.ac.uk/bandolier/band84/MMR.html> (**Figure** 1.3).

♦ A video, produced by the US Center for Disease Control and Prevention 'Safer Healthier Children: A Brief Introduction to Childhood Vaccines' <http://www.cdc.gov/nip/vaccine/ABCs/vac-video.htm>

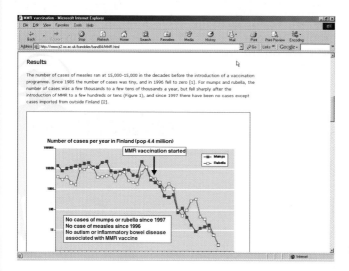

Figure 1.3 *Benefits of MMR – as published by Bandolier*

Conclusion

Having briefly demonstrated the potential of the Internet, we need to consider how we can find information relevant to our specific needs and circumstances. Before we do this, however, we need to examine how we 'log on' on to the Internet and use the key Internet tools – namely the Web browser and email.

Web browsing and email

Box 2.1   Chapter objectives

♦ Introduce the concept of Web browsing.

♦ Discuss how to use a Web browser effectively, looking at issues such as bookmarks, filtering content, and online security.

♦ Provide a beginner's guide to using email.

♦ Highlight a number of email-related issues, such as computer viruses and spam and discuss how these can be managed.

Introduction

Figures from the Office of National Statistics show that in the second quarter of 2004, 52% of households in the UK (12.8 million) could access the Internet from home, compared with just 9% (2.2 million) in the same quarter of 1998.

Although part of this growth in connectivity can be ascribed to curiosity and a wish not to be left behind in the information revolution, repeated surveys on why individuals are connecting to the Internet show two recurring themes. First, there is a desire to use the Web to gain access to information sources and services, such as online banking and shopping. Beyond this, the second reason given for seeking Internet connectivity is a wish to be able to communicate cheaply and easily with friends and colleagues throughout the world. To achieve this, email is recognised as the communications tool of choice.

In this chapter we will discuss Web browsing and email, focusing in particular on how to make effective use of the software to access these services. We will also highlight some of the risks of Internet connectivity – such as email viruses and unwanted mail (spam) – and discuss how these can be managed.

Web browser

To be able to view a Web site – such as <http://www.bbc.co.uk> – you need a Web browser. A browser is simply a piece of software (like a word processing programme) that is installed on your computer that you use when you want to access the Internet.

To open your web browser, you will need to point your mouse to the browser 'icon' on your desktop (see **Figure 2.1**) and 'double click' on it. Icons are the small logos used to indicate which applications you have installed on your computer. The relevant folder/program/application can then be opened-up by 'double clicking' on it using your mouse.

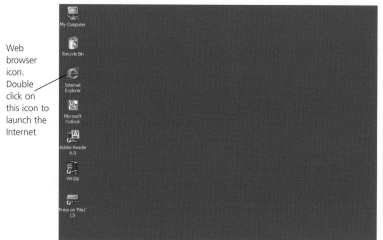

Web browser icon. Double click on this icon to launch the Internet

Figure 2.1
Typical desktop showing the Web browser icon

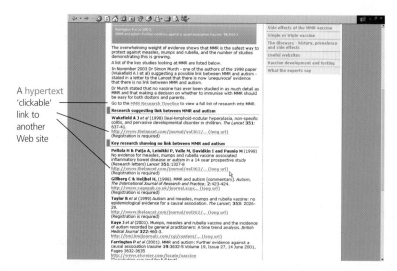

A hypertext 'clickable' link to another Web site

Figure 2.2
Web page – with hypertext, clickable links to related documents on other Web sites

In addition to being able to display a particular page, Web browsers can also link to other pages and sites – irrespective of their physical location – through the use of hypertext. For example, the 'MMR – The Facts' Web site <http://www.mmrthefacts.nhs.uk/> highlights various research papers that discuss whether there is a link between MMR and autism. Rather than copy the data from the various sites (*Lancet, BMJ* etc.) the MMR site is simply connected by hypertext links to the original data (**Figure 2.2**).

Although today there are a number of Web browsers available, the market is dominated by Microsoft's Internet Explorer and Netscape's Navigator. Both are available free of charge and can be acquired either on CD-ROM (distributed by Internet Service Providers or magazines that focus on the Internet) or directly from the Internet.

Using the browser – the basics

Irrespective of which browser you use, all support common features that can be accessed through the standard toolbar. **Table 2.1** provides a summary of these features.

Bookmarks and favourites

As you start to explore the Internet there will undoubtedly be some sites you will wish to return to. MEDLINE (see Chapter 8), for example, is a key resource that you may wish to access on a regular basis. Although you can re-key the Web address <http://www.ncbi.nlm.nih.gov/PubMed> every time you wish to access this site, it makes more sense to use the Bookmark/Favorite feature within the Web browser to record this (and other) URLs. (Note: Netscape uses the term Bookmarks, whilst Microsoft prefers Favorites.)

Once you have 'bookmarked' a site, you can revisit it by calling up the bookmarked list and clicking on the relevant site (**Figure 2.3**).

Security

There has been a great deal of concern about the security of the Internet and in particular, is it wise to transmit your personal details or credit card numbers over this network? Although *any* system is open to abuse, if the Web site you are accessing uses a secure system you can be reasonably assured that your transaction will not be tampered with.

When accessing a secure site, users of Internet Explorer will be presented with an information box informing them of this change in status (by default Web pages are not secure) and a locked padlock will appear on the bottom of the browser window.

> *Always check that a site is secure before submitting personal details. If in doubt, always err on the side of caution.*

Top Tip

Table 2.1 Web browser – toolbar functions

In the following table function commands appear in the form **menu name → command**. Thus, **File → Save**, means open the file menu and select the save option.

Ctrl refers to the Control key, located at the bottom left hand side of the keyboard.

Where commands are browser specific IE will be used to indicate Internet Explorer and NS to signify Netscape's Navigator.

Toolbar option	Function
Back & Forward	Use these keys to go back (and forward) to Web pages previously accessed.
Stop	Use to stop loading the current page – a useful function if the page is big (in terms of the number of images etc.) and/or slow.
Refresh	Sometimes a page will be corrupted as it is transmitted. This will be evident in either missing text or images. Using the Refresh key forces the browser to go back to the original server and re-request the page.
Home	The Home page is the page the browser defaults to when the application is first opened. This should be set to open up the page you consider to be most useful. A web search engine (Chapter 3) may be a suitable candidate. IE – Tools → Internet Options → General → Home Page NS – Edit → Preferences → Navigator → Home Page
Search	Use this button to connect to an Internet search engine.
Address/Location	This is where the Web address (known as a URL) of every page is displayed. This address/location box can also be used to enter any Web page you wish to access. Throughout this book you will see Web addresses in the form <http://webaddress.suffix>. If you want to access any of these pages simply enter the full address as cited in the address/location box. If you prefer, the http:// prefix can be omitted.
History	The History function can be used to view previously accessed pages. IE – File → Work Offline. Click on the History icon (or press Ctrl-H) NS – File → Offline → Work Offline, then Communicator → Tools → History (or press Ctrl-H) Any page in the History file can be selected and viewed.
Multiple windows	Use Ctrl-N to open up multiple browser windows.

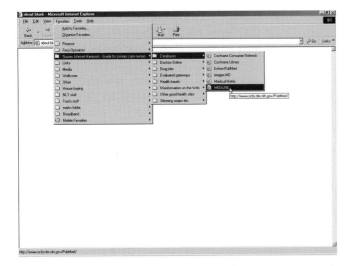

Figure 2.3 *Bookmarks – arranged hierarchically for easy access*

Filtering content

There may be occasions when you want to filter the information that can be found on the Internet. For example, the easy availability of pornography on the Internet is well known and if children are going to use the Internet it is advisable to introduce some form of filtering.

Although you can **download** various content-filtering software programs from the Internet, both the leading browsers have in-built filtering facilities that filter material based on agreed international standards and personal preferences.

The mechanism behind content filtering is very simple. At the browser level you determine the level of filtering you wish to employ, in categories such as language, sex and violence (**Figure 2.4**). At the other end of the chain,

Internet options is under the 'Tools' menu

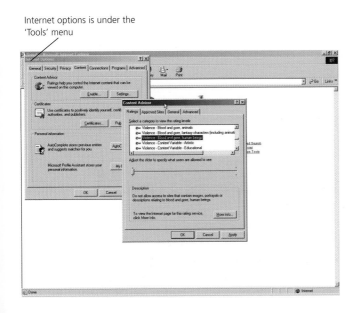

Figure 2.4
Implementing filters in Internet Explorer

Web authors embed tags into a Web page to indicate the level of nudity or violence on a specific page. Once the level of filtering has been defined, access to any Web page whose content exceeds that level is denied.

A number of organisations have drawn up codes of practice for 'safe browsing' and parents interested in this topic are advised to read the one developed by the Internet Watch Foundation, available at: <http://www.internetwatch.org.uk/safe/tip.htm>

Email

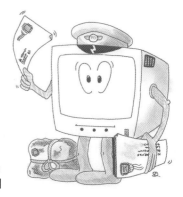

Despite the attention that is afforded to the Web, the desire to be able to send and receive emails is a key motivating factor for seeking Internet access. Email is fast, virtually cost-free and highly efficient. It can be used to send both text and binary files (word-processing files, spreadsheets, images, etc.) and once you start using it in earnest, the idea of writing and posting a letter (known as 'snail mail') or sending a fax seems somewhat labour intensive and inconvenient.

Email – the basics

To send and receive emails you require email software. Typically, this will already be installed on your computer; with Microsoft's Outlook and Outlook Express being the most popular email programs.

Irrespective of which email program you use, all support common features that can be accessed through the standard toolbar (**Figure 2.5**). **Table 2.2** provides a summary of these features.

Clicking on this button will forward on a message and all its attachments

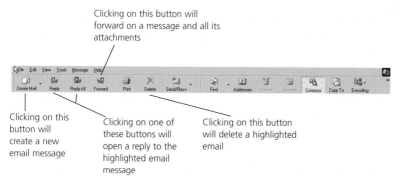

Clicking on this button will create a new email message

Clicking on one of these buttons will open a reply to the highlighted email message

Clicking on this button will delete a highlighted email

Figure 2.5 *Outlook Express (email) toolbar*

Table 2.2   Email – toolbar functions

Toolbar option	Function
Compose message	Opens a window for you to compose your email message.
To; cc, Bcc	In this box you enter the email address of the person you wish to communicate with. Via the *cc* option you can copy the message to another person or group of people. *Bcc* (blind carbon copy) allows you to copy the message to a third party (or groups of people) without the original recipients (as identified in the *To*: section) being aware of this.
Reply/Reply to all	One of the powerful and attractive features of email is that you can reply to any message by a single keystroke. You do not need to bother keying in an email address – the email software will do that for you and as the original message is included in the reply, answers can be inserted immediately adjacent to any question.
	If a message had been copied to others, the *Reply to All* option will send your one response to all recipients.
Forward	Use this option to forward any received email to anyone else you think might be interested in it.
Address book	As email addresses are invariably forgettable, it makes sense to keep a record of them in an electronic address book. Addresses in this book can be copied into the *To*, *cc* and *Bcc* boxes.
Attachments	In addition to any text message you compose you can also attach other files to your email. These may include documents you have created using a word processing package, spreadsheets, or images.

Attachments

In addition to being able to send messages to friends and colleagues throughout the world, email also supports the use of attachments. As the name implies, an attachment is a digital file you attach to the email. This digital file may take the form of a word-processed document, an image or even a video clip.

Attachments – because they are binary files rather than simple text files – can also carry computer viruses. Consequently, before opening any attachment it is good practice to use a virus checker (see over).

Email conventions

Unlike the telephone where your tone of voice adds meaning, or in a letter where a scented envelope would speak volumes, email users can only determine meaning through the typed word. In an attempt to minimise the chance of being misunderstood various keyboard-codes have been devised. For example, to indicate that your comment is meant to be taken in jest the ;-) code is used. [If you tip your head through 90° you should get the idea of someone winking at you!]

You should also be aware that once you have sent an email you have no control over how it may be used in the future. It may, for example, be forwarded to other individuals, or even distributed to whole groups of people via discussion lists and newsgroups.

> *Always re-read your emails before sending them to make sure your meaning is clear. Once a mail has been sent – it cannot be retrieved!*

Top Tip

Viruses

Another aspect to consider when using email is the potential threat of contracting a computer virus. A virus is a piece of software that has been written to secretly enter your computer system and 'infect' your files. Some viruses are benign and will not harm your computer, while others are destructive and can damage or destroy your data.

The main distribution medium for computer viruses is email. The beauty of email, in the eyes of the people who write these viruses, is the ease by which the virus can be spread. As soon as anyone receives an infected email, all new mail that is sent from that computer carries the virus. This way the virus can continue to replicate itself.

To ensure that your computer does not become infected, you need to install some anti-virus software. There are a number of suitable products on the market, many of which can be found at <http://dmoz.org/Computers/ Security/Malicious_Software/Viruses/Products>. Once installed you need to subscribe to an update service to ensure that your system remains protected at all times.

Spam

In recent years, one of the biggest problems Internet users have had to deal with is unwanted mail – spam. Indeed, recent research suggests that over 60% of all email traffic is now spam.

Typically, spam mail offers the recipient the opportunity to purchase something, such as drugs (eg Viagra), university degrees, software, pornography, etc at low cost (or even free of charge), or participate in 'money-making, risk-free' schemes. In reality, it is doubtful whether goods and services offered this way really exist, whilst get-rich quick schemes should be considered as works of fiction.

More recently, spam attacks have tried to induce recipients to disclose their Internet banking user names and passwords. This spam is perpetrated by sending an email that *appears* to come from a legitimate source (eg Barclays Bank). Unfortunately some people have believed these mails to be *bona fide*, only to find later that their bank account has been cleared of all funds.

Box 2.2 highlights some of the steps you can take to minimise and manage spam mail.

Box 2.2   Managing spam mail

♦ Don't ever reply to spam mail – as it will simply confirm to the spammer that the email address is valid.

♦ Value your email address as you would your phone number.

♦ Consider setting up an alternative email account solely for the purpose of writing to newsgroups or buying online. Although this account may be subject to spam, your other, primary account (because the address is not in the public domain) will remain relatively spam-free.

♦ If your email software has spam-blocking features, switch them on. **Figure 2.6** shows the Junk mail controls in Thunderbird <http://www.mozilla.org/products/thunderbird/>.

♦ If your email program cannot deal with the spam, consider installing a dedicated anti-spam program, such as Mailwasher <http://www.mailwasher.net/>.

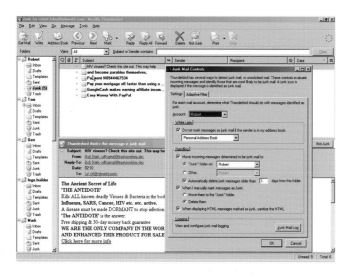

Figure 2.6   *Managing spam – using the Thunderbird email software*

Conclusion

Once you have set up and experimented with your Web browser and email programs the potential of the Internet begins to become apparent. To help you exploit this potential we must now look beyond the basics and consider how you can search the Internet and find information relevant to your needs.

Searching the Web

CHAPTER 3

Box 3.1   Chapter objectives

♦ Highlight the different approaches you can use to search the Internet.

♦ Provide a tutorial-like guide to Internet searching.

♦ Demonstrate, through worked examples, how you can search the Internet to find information specific to your needs.

♦ Provide tips on how to develop effective search strategies.

Introduction

Users new to the Internet are often surprised by how easy it is to search for information. All Web browsers have 'Search' buttons on their toolbars (see Chapter 2), which, when clicked on, direct you to a Web site where you can key-in your search terms to identify relevant Web pages.

While this method of searching is easy, its effectiveness is more questionable. For example, a Google search for the phrase 'pain control' identifies over 6,000,000 pages. Undoubtedly, some of the resources suggested are highly useful – the information on pain control provided by the US National Cancer Institute <http://cancernet.nci.nih.gov/> being a case in point. Other resources, however, such as Web sites that focus on the heavy metal band of the same name <http://www.pain-control.co.uk/> are obviously irrelevant. Sifting the results to sort the wheat from the chaff can be time-consuming.

This chapter, therefore, seeks to provide a tutorial-like guide to *effective* Internet searching. Specifically, we will highlight a number of search tools and provide tips to help ensure that whatever topic you are researching on the Web, the information you find will be relevant to your needs.

Search tools

In December 1993 an email message sent to the Internet newsgroup <news://comp.infosystems.www> included a list of *all* the Web sites that were available on the Internet: the list detailed just 623 sites. Some 12 years later, the number of Web sites is estimated to exceed 40 million, whilst the number of *pages* on the Web is in excess of eight billion.

With so much information available, the practice of sending lists of Web sites to relevant newsgroups is now somewhat futile. Fortunately, various tools have been developed to help people navigate through this mass of data and discover information relevant to their interests.

Searching the Web typically involves the use of the following tools:

♦ search services
♦ directory services
♦ evaluated gateway services.

This chapter considers each of these approaches and, through worked examples, shows how a specific query was answered. These can subsequently be used as templates for any information search you may wish to undertake.

Search services: an overview

Before we discuss the specifics of searching the Internet using a service like Google, it is useful to have some understanding of how these services function.

In simple terms a computer program (known as a robot or spider) crawls the Internet in search of Web pages, images, videos, etc. When the robot program finds a Web resource it copies all the words and images that are on that page and adds them to its database. As most Web pages have links to other pages the robot can follow those links and retrieve yet more pages. This process continues indefinitely. Thus, when you perform a search, you are simply running a query against a database of Web pages.

For your Internet searching to be effective – namely, to find a small number of highly appropriate resources – you need to plan your search strategy. Detailed below are a number of top tips to help you develop effective search strategies.

At present there are approximately 12 popular search tools and all have their own strengths and weaknesses. In this section, however, we are going to limit our discussion to the search service offered by Google.

Top Tip

◆ **Clarify your search**

If you are simply looking for information on a single concept – migraine, asthma, etc – then you have little choice other than to undertake a very simple single-word search. If, however, you are more interested in, for example, the use of acupuncture in managing migraine or the relationship between air pollution and asthma, then adding these terms to your search query will help identify the more relevant sites.

◆ **Be aware of synonyms**

Consider using synonyms to ensure that all relevant pages are retrieved. For example, pages that provide information about breast cancer may use alternative terms such as 'breast neoplasms' or 'breast tumours'. If you wanted to find all pages relevant to this condition you would need to use all the synonyms in your search.

◆ **Be alert to variants in spelling**

Similarly, be alert to variants in the way some terms are spelt. Continuing with the example cited above you would need to search for both 'breast tumour' and 'breast tumor'(English and US spellings) if your search were to identify all relevant pages.

◆ **Think laterally**

When trying to find the answer to a specific question try to think where the answer may have been published – rather than just key-in your question. For example, if you were trying to identify official statistics about the incidence of BSE/CJD in the United Kingdom it is likely that the Department of Health would publish this type of data. Use Google to identify the Web address of this site.

Google

<http://www.google.com>

With a reported search index of more that 8 billion Web pages (November 2004) Google provides the biggest and most comprehensive search service.

To find relevant Web sites using Google you simply enter terms in the query box and press the *Google Search* button. The interface is clear, uncluttered and advertising-free. Once a search has been executed – which is remarkably fast given the size of the index it has to search – you are told how many Web pages contain information relevant to the query, and are provided with a list of these pages (**Figure 3.1**).

What really differentiates Google from the other search sites, however, is the way it ranks the results – so that the most relevant site appears at (or near) the top of your list. Google achieves this by employing a technique known as PageRank. PageRank takes into account how many other sites link to a specific page, and who is making the link. This way, popular and highly cited Web sites rise to the top of the list.

Web addresses are typed in here   Search terms are typed in here – the
query box – and then the big 'search'
button to the right is clicked on

Number of websites found
containing information on
diabetes

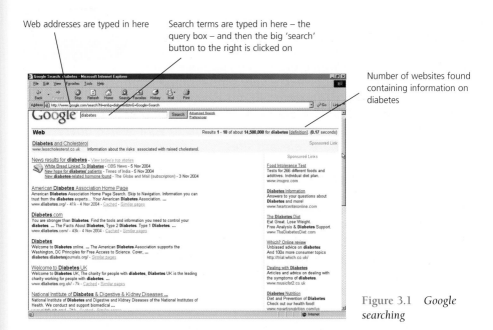

Figure 3.1   *Google
searching*

For example, a Google search for Web sites that discuss diabetes clearly demonstrates the power of this ranking technology. Although such a simple search generated numerous hits – more than 14 million Web pages have information on this topic – at the top of this list were the Web sites of the American Diabetes Association, Diabetes UK, and the National Institute of Diabetes and Digestive and Kidney Diseases of the National Institutes of Health. All three sites are highly regarded and anyone looking for an authoritative overview of the disease will find these sites particularly useful.

Google also has an advanced search page <http://www.google.com/advanced_search> that supports a number of useful options, including the facility to limit material to a particular language, and the opportunity to include (or exclude) pages from a defined domain. This latter option is very useful if, for example, you want to restrict a search to pages that are in the '.uk' domain.

Box 3.2 provides a step-by-step worked example of how Google was used to find information about some recently published research.

Other search services

Table 3.1 highlights a number of other search services.

Directory services

The second approach to finding information on the Internet is to search (or browse) through one of the many Web directories that are now online. These directories attempt to classify Web resources into meaningful subject groupings.

Box 3.2   Searching using Google: a worked example

Question

A recent newspaper article made reference to a study that regular tea drinkers may have better memories and are less likely to develop Alzheimer's disease. Can the Internet be used to help identify this research?

Answer & Methodology

Although the databases of medical research (MEDLINE, CINAHL, etc – see Chapter 8) would be the best way to identify the peer-reviewed medical literature on this topic, in this example we will assume that we are simply looking for general information about the effectiveness of tea in improving memory and minimising the risk of Alzheimer's.

We will also assume that we are looking for information published within the past three months and, if possible, for information published in the United Kingdom.

The methodology for this search is detailed below:

1. Point your browser at Google. As we want to do a reasonably sophisticated search, go to the advanced search page <http://www.google.com/advanced_search>.

2. In the search box type in a search concept. In this example, enter the following: **Alzheimer's tea memory**.
    [These are the three key concepts.]

3. From the pull-down menus (**Figure 3.2**) specify that pages should be written in **English**, have been published within the past three months and should form part of the **.uk** domain.

4. Google returns with a ranked list of over 1300 relevant pages. Resources identified include a recent news articles on the BBC Web site an article in the Guardian newspaper and information on this subject from the Alzheimer's Society (**Figure 3.3**).

5. On following the link to the BBC article, you are provided with a brief overview of the research and given links to related Web sites, including the *Physiotherapy Journal* where the original research was published.

Comment

This search demonstrates the power of Google. Despite the size of the Google database, this well-defined search returned highly relevant Web sites within a matter of seconds.

Typically, Web directories are also hierarchical in nature – a feature that allows you to 'drill down' to more specific subjects.

The ability to identify Internet resources from a broad subject base also negates the need to search for highly specific terms. This can be a particularly useful feature if you are new to a subject and unsure of the best or most appropriate terminology.

Table 3.1 Other search services

Service	URL	Key feature
AltaVista	\<http://www.altavista.com/>	♦ Good at searching for formats such as video clips and audio (MP3) files.
AskJeeves	\<http://www.ask.com/>	♦ Good for 'natural language searching.'
Teoma	\<http://www.teoma.com/>	♦ Uses a ranking system based on the number of same-subject pages that reference a known site.

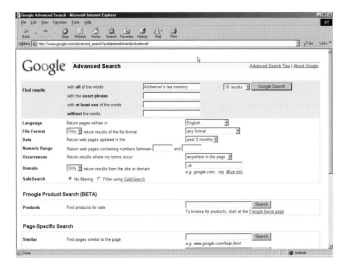

Figure 3.2 *Google – Advanced searching*

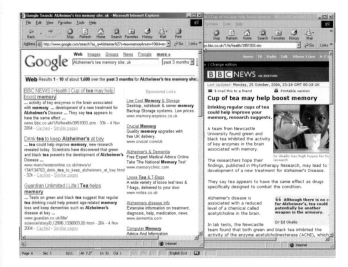

Figure 3.3. *Results from Google Advanced search*

Described below is the Open Directory – the single biggest Web directory.

Open Directory Project
<http://dmoz.org>

The Open Directory Project (ODP) is described as 'the largest, most comprehensive human-edited directory of the Web, constructed and maintained by a vast, global community of volunteer editors'. These volunteers, who have an interest in or knowledge of a specific subject, identify useful Web sites for the benefit of non-experts. At the time of writing, the ODP had some 65,000 editors who had indexed more than four million sites, in over 590,000 subject categories.

The easiest way to use this service is to search the entire directory. For example, a search for 'family planning' will lead you to resources in various parts of the subject hierarchy such as:

◆ Health: Reproductive Health
◆ Health: Reproductive Health: Birth Control: Natural Family Planning
◆ Society: Issues: Family Planning

On navigating to the first section identified (Health: Reproductive Health), you are directed to a number of sites that discuss all aspects of family planning, as well as related concepts, such as infertility and sexually transmitted diseases. If the concepts are too broad, you can select a narrower subject heading, such as 'Birth Control', and even more specific concepts, such as 'Barrier Methods', 'Emergency Contraception' or 'Hormonal Methods'.

Type your search term here

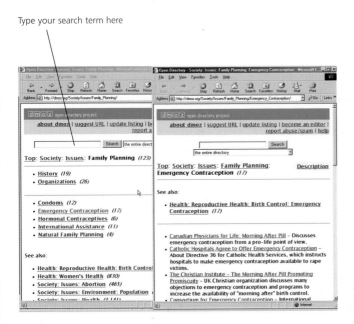

Figure 3.4   *Open Directory Project*

At each subject-level a list of relevant Web sites is provided and to help you determine which are the most appropriate to your information needs, a brief one-line description is given (**Figure 3.4**).

Box 3.3 provides a step-by-step worked example of how the Open Directory was used to find information about primary care nursing.

Box 3.3   Searching using the Open Directory: a worked example

Question

A nurse working in primary care wants to know what is available on the Internet for this group of health professionals.

Answer & Methodology

As this is a very general search, Google and other search services would be of little use. Although you could search for 'primary care nursing' – this would only find Web pages that contained this term and would therefore overlook potential relevant resources, such as those that dealt with childhood vaccination, travel health, etc. Consequently, a more effective approach is to use a Web directory service, like the Open Directory.

The methodology and results are described below.

1. Point your browser at the Open Directory <http://dmoz.org/>.

2. As there is no obvious single search term – community nursing, nursing in primary care, public health nurse, etc. – we decide to *browse* the directory.

3. From the top-level '**Health**' heading we navigate to '**Nursing**' and then to the more specific heading '**Nursing Specialities**'. Here we are presented with various headings, such as '**Critical Care**', '**Perioperative Nursing**', '**Triage**' and '**Community Health**'.

4. The latter concept sounds promising, and from this page Web links are provided to resources such as the *British Journal of Community Care Nursing* <http://www.britishjournalofcommunitynursing.com/> and the *Journal of Community Nursing* <http://www.jcn.co.uk/>.

5. The Open Directory also provides links to more specific directory sections – Community Health Associations – as well as related (and broader) concepts such as 'Patient Education'.

Comment

Although the resources identified here do not represent the totality of Internet resources for primary care nurses, they nevertheless provide nurses working in this specialty with an excellent starting point.

Other directory services

Table 3.2 highlights a number of other directory services.

Table 3.2 Other directory services

Service	URL	Key feature
Yahoo!	<http://uk.yahoo.com/>	♦ The first Web directory – still highly regarded.
LookSmart	<http://www.looksmart.com/>	♦ In addition to categorising the Web by subject, LookSmart also provides access to content from thousands of online periodicals.
Yell	<http://www.yell.com/>	♦ BT's 'Yellow pages' – both searchable and browsable.

Evaluated gateway services

The third way to find health resources on the Internet is to use an evaluated subject gateway. In many ways these look and function much like the Web directories. The key difference, however, is that these directories only list sites that meet defined quality standards.

Because each resource in the directory has to be checked for quality, the number of Web sites indexed by these services is inevitably relatively small. Consequently, although these services will direct you to Internet sites of high quality, their coverage can be somewhat limited.

Described below is the NMAP – the Internet gateway for Nursing, Midwifery and Allied Health Professions.

NMAP
<http://nmap.ac.uk>

NMAP, developed by information specialists and subject experts based in the UK, is a gateway to evaluated Internet resources aimed at students, researchers and practitioners in the health and medical sciences.

The 3500 Web resources described in this database can be both searched and browsed. Recognising the power of browsing, the NMAP team have developed an interface that allows you to browse the database by MeSH subject headings. This facility allows you to select broader and narrower concepts, thus facilitating more precise and focused browsing. For example, on selecting the MeSH term 'Immunisation' you are given the opportunity to elect a more specific term, 'Vaccination', a broader term, 'Communicable Disease Control' or a related term such as 'Infection Control'.

Box 3.4 provides a step-by-step worked example of how NMAP was used to find information relating to the management of leg ulcers.

Box 3.4   Searching using NMAP: a worked example

Question

A primary care nurse wishes to find some high-quality information on the management of leg ulcers.

Answer & Methodology

Although either of the search tools discussed previously (Google and Open Directory) could be used to answer this question, as the focus of this search is to find a number of high-quality Internet resources it makes sense to use an evaluated gateway service, like NMAP.

The methodology and results are described below.

1. Point your browser at the NMAP gateway <http://nmap.ac.uk>.

2. Select the '**Browse**' option (located on the toolbar) and select '**RCN Headings**'. Although these subject headings do not support broader and narrower terms (useful for expanding or refining a search), as they were devised by the Royal College of Nursing the terms used have a UK-focus (and meaning).

3. From the A–Z alphabetical listing, navigate to '**L**' and from the list of terms, select **Leg Ulcers** (**Figure 3.5**).

4. At this page a number of relevant sounding resources are identified including 'Clinical guidelines on the management of leg ulcers' (from the RCN) and a study, published in July 2004, that compared the effectiveness of two different compression bandages for the healing of venous leg ulcers.

Comment

This example demonstrates that evaluated gateway services represent an excellent way to find relevant and authoritative information.

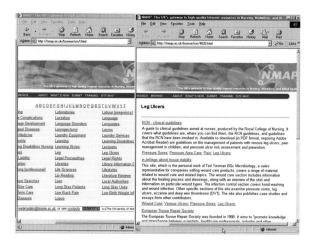

Figure 3.5   *Browsing NMAP – and search results*

Other search services

Table 3.3 highlights a number of other evaluated gateways.

Table 3.3   Other evaluated gateway services

Service	URL	Key feature
OMNI	<http://omni.ac.uk/>	♦ The most authoritative UK health/medical gateway service
MedlinePlus	<http://medlineplus.gov>	♦ Developed by the US National Library of Medicine, this is an excellent guide to some of the best health sites on the Internet.
Health on the Net	<http://www.hon.ch/>	♦ Provides both lay users and medical professionals with a guide to reliable sources of healthcare information on the Internet.

Assessing quality

The quality of health information on the Internet is extremely variable. Try using Google and searching for, say, 'cancer'. You will find that you can move seamlessly from authoritative sites like Cancernet <http://www.nci.nih.gov> and OncoLink <http://cancer.med.upenn.edu>, through to highly dubious ones that claim, for example, that all cancers are caused by 'a parasite' – if you kill the parasite, then the cancer is cured and this can be achieved by the simple use of a 'zapper'.

Although it would be wonderful if one of the biggest killers in the Western world could be defeated so simply, there is, unfortunately, no evidence that this treatment has any effect on any form of cancer. Moreover, although in itself the Zapper will do little harm, there is a real danger that some patients will try this method before, or instead of, seeking appropriate care. The consequence of this approach may be fatal.

Misinformation of this kind is not the only problem that besets the health-information seeker. Web sites that are highly biased and only present one side of the argument are another concern, as is the ability to buy drugs and medical devices that may be unregulated, unproven and potentially dangerous. In Chapter 9 we will provide examples of these types of sites.

Conclusion

This chapter has demonstrated the different methodologies and tools you can use to find information on the Internet. Armed with this knowledge you can now search the Internet effectively, secure in the knowledge that if it is on the Web – you will be able to find it.

The medical Web: starting points

CHAPTER 4

Box 4.1 Chapter objectives

♦ Identify a number of high-quality Web sites on topics of general interest to UK nurses in primary care.

♦ Provide a starting point for further exploration.

Introduction

There are many organisations that provide information useful to health professionals via the Web, and the number of organisations with a Web presence is constantly increasing. In this chapter, we have identified a selection of high-quality resources relating to *general* topics of particular relevance to nurses in primary care.

UK Government sites

Department of Health

<http://www.dh.gov.uk/Home/fs/en>

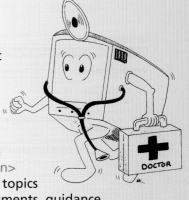

This official government site is primarily aimed at health and social care professionals, as well as academics and the public (**Figure 4.1**).

The Department of Health (DH) is responsible for setting health and social care policy in England. The Policy and Guidance section of the site <http://www.dh.gov.uk/PolicyAndGuidance/fs/en> contains subsections on a comprehensive range of topics in healthcare and social care, including policy documents, guidance on implementation, non-clinical guidance, newsletters, links and other resources. A subsection on Human Resources and Training covers topics, such as pay policy, working conditions and personal and professional development.

Click here to find out about DH publications

Type in a search term here to see if it is covered on the DH website

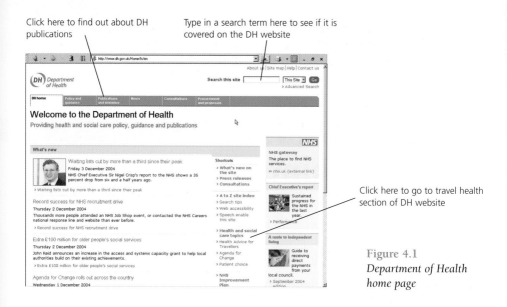

Click here to go to travel health section of DH website

Figure 4.1
Department of Health home page

A news page <http://www.dh.gov.uk/NewsHome/fs/en> provides the latest health news released from the Department, what's new on the DH Web site, speeches, events and links to recent and archived press releases and bulletins.

Almost all current and many old DH publications, including statistical reports, surveys, press releases, circulars and legislation, are available in electronic form on the site. The publications library can be searched or browsed by category. Hard copies of most documents can be ordered free of charge.

National electronic Library for Health (NeLH)
<http://www.nelh.nhs.uk/>

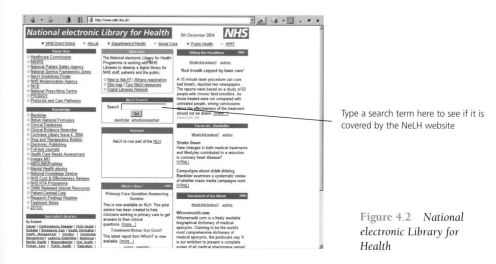

Type a search term here to see if it is covered by the NeLH website

Figure 4.2 *National electronic Library for Health*

The National electronic Library for Health (NeLH) is a gateway to a large number of electronic resources targeted primarily at NHS staff, and aims 'to provide clinicians with access to the best current know-how and knowledge to support healthcare-related decisions' (**Figure 4.2**).

A wealth of information includes links to National Service Frameworks, protocols and care pathways, guidance and guidelines, key documents, and commentaries on news stories. Other features are links to Specialist Libraries, and to Professional Portals including a Nurse portal at <http://www.nelh.nhs.uk/nurse/> and a Primary Care portal at <http://www.nelh.nhs.uk/primarycare/>. (The NeLH is in the final stages of commissioning a new Primary Care Information Service, due to be launched later this year.)

Most of the resources on the site are freely available, but some (including all resources in the NHS Core Content Collection) are available only via a PC connected to the NHSnet, or to eligible users with an Athens username and password. NHS staff can register at the NeLH site for an Athens account.

NHS Direct Online
<http://www.nhsdirect.nhs.uk/>

NHS Direct Online is a Web gateway to high-quality health information and advice for residents in England. It is unique in being supported by a 24-hour nurse advice and information helpline (0845 4647). An online health information enquiry service is also available for users who are unable to find the information they require on the Web site. (It can only provide information about named health conditions.)

The site includes a Health Encyclopaedia <http://www.nhsdirect.nhs.uk/resourceindex.asp> (**Figure 4.3**) that can be searched or browsed (alphabetically or by subject area) to find information on medical

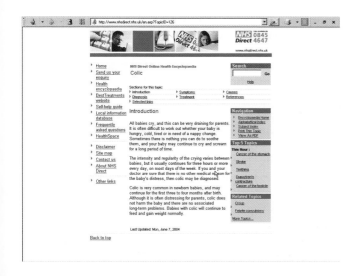

Figure 4.3   *NHS Direct Online - Health Encyclopaedia*

conditions, tests and treatments. A Self Help Guide <http://www.nhsdirect.nhs.uk/selfhelp/index.asp> covers the most common symptoms which people call NHS Direct about for advice.

The site links to the NHS in England site <http://www.nhs.uk/england/> for information about local and national NHS services, including contact details for doctors, dentists, opticians and pharmacies.

NHS Gateway

<http://www.nhs.uk/>

This is the official gateway to NHS organisations on the Internet: it provides access to a wide range of health-related Web sites, including links to all of the NHS sites mentioned above, as well as to information about how the NHS works and finding and registering for NHS services.

A section on working for the NHS includes links to information about careers <http://www.nhscareers.nhs.uk/> and to job vacancies <http://www.jobs.nhs.uk/>; the jobs site was shortlisted as a finalist for the National Online Recruitment Awards.

> *Save time by registering with the site, and sign up to receive 'Jobs by Email'.*

Top Tip

PRODIGY

http://www.prodigy.nhs.uk/Nurse/

PRODIGY is a source of clinical knowledge, based on the best available evidence, about the common conditions and symptoms managed in primary care. It was developed, and is updated by, a team at the Sowerby Centre for Health Informatics at Newcastle. It covers around 170 guidance topics for both acute and chronic illnesses, and is structured to support both decision-making in the consultation and learning outside of the consultation.

On the Web site PRODIGY guidance is available as full text documents, quick reference guides and Patient Information Leaflets (PILs).

A selection of the guidance is also represented by 'Quick reference guides' <http://www.prodigy.nhs.uk/QuickReferenceGuides/>, which summarise the key management options within the guidance, providing concise supporting information and prescription details. They are usually only one or two sides of A4 when printed, intended to be handy desktop guides. (The range is constantly being expanded; the intention is eventually to have a quick reference guide for each guidance topic.)

Registration is not necessary to use the site, but users are encouraged to do so to help the authors to 'customise the site to match the needs of our users'.

UK Nursing sites

Royal College of Nursing

<http://www.rcn.org.uk>

The Royal College of Nursing represents nurses and nursing in the UK. Their Web site includes information about the RCN, details of forthcoming events, campaigns and conferences, and news. An extensive range of information about nursing includes courses, pay, clinical guidelines and other publications, and the history of nursing.

Some areas of the site are available to members only. Within the RCN membership cost, you can join any three of the specialist forums; the RCN Travel Health Forum is found within the primary care and public health section at <http://www.rcn.org.uk/specialisms/primarycare.php>.

Nursing and Midwifery Council

<http://www.nmc-uk.org/>

The Nursing and Midwifery Council was 'set up by Parliament to ensure nurses, midwives and health visitors provide high standards of care to their patients and clients'. This site is structured into areas providing information for practitioners, the public, employers and job seekers. The Practitioners' area <http://www.nmc-uk.org/nmc/main/home.html> includes information on registration, quality assurance, consultation, advice, publications and links to other useful Web sites.

The Community Practitioners and Health Visitors Association (CPHVA)

<http://www.amicus-cphva.org/>

The CPHVA website has been created to make information about the organisation and its work available online, and to provide a gateway to other sites which provide information on community nursing, public health and primary health care. The 'home' area, which includes a brief section on practice nursing, is freely available. A members' area, which contains more detailed information, can be accessed only by CPHVA members.

Framework for Nursing in General Practice

<http://www.show.scot.nhs.uk/sehd/practicenursing/index.htm>

In September 2004, following consultation with nurses, the Scottish Executive launched a new *Framework for Nursing in General Practice.* The Web site sets out the purpose of the framework, shares current work in progress and seeks contributions on good practice and issues in the field of practice nursing.

Nurses Network

<http://www.nursesnetwork.co.uk/>

Nurses Network is an online nurses community 'devoted to bringing nurses together', developed by UK qualified nurses. It aims to provide a forum for communication and access to information, advice and news. The site is arranged into 'departments', including Practice Nurses. Other features include links to other relevant resources, chat forums and news.

UK Patient sites

NetDoctor

<http://www.netdoctor.co.uk/>

NetDoctor.co.uk is 'a collaboration between committed doctors, healthcare professionals, information specialists and patients who believe that medical practice should be based on quality-assessed information and, wherever possible, on the basis of the principles of evidence-based medicine'. Acknowledging that an increasing number of patients now seek out critical medical information on the Internet, their aim is to provide it in a clearly expressed, intelligible form.

This detailed and informative site includes information on diseases and conditions, examinations and procedures, medicines, news stories and special features. A team of GPs and health advisers provide a 24-hour online 'Ask the doctor' service; the questions and answers are archived and made available in a searchable and browsable form.

Patient UK

<http://www.patient.co.uk/>

Patient UK aims to be 'a reliable and comprehensive source of health and disease information, mainly aimed at the UK general public, but of interest to all.' A Web directory includes links to health and illness related Web sites, which have been reviewed by GPs. These cover primarily UK sites (as the authors feel that residents in the UK prefer to obtain health information from UK sources), but include selected overseas sites.

Other valuable features include: a directory of nearly 2000 UK patient support organisations (**Figure 4.4**), self help groups, health and disease information providers; over 600 patient information leaflets on health and disease; and over 800 leaflets on medicines and drugs.

International sites

World Health Organization

<http://www.who.int/en/>

The World Health Organization is the United Nations specialised agency for health. WHO's objective, as set out in its Constitution, is 'the attainment by all peoples of the highest possible level of health', defined as 'state of

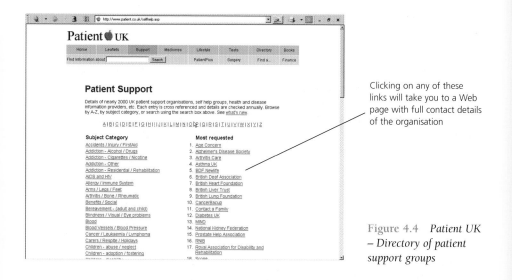

Clicking on any of these links will take you to a Web page with full contact details of the organisation

Figure 4.4   *Patient UK – Directory of patient support groups*

complete physical, mental and social well-being and not merely the absence of disease or infirmity.'

The health topics pages <http://www.who.int/topics/en/> contain links to WHO projects, initiatives, activities, information products, and contacts, organised by health and development topics. A series of country-specific pages includes the UK at <http://www.who.int/countries/gbr/en/>. The site also provides access to WHO publications, press releases, and links to other WHO sites.

The section on International Travel and Health <http://www.who.int/ith/> will be referred to in more detail in Chapter 7.

International Council of Nurses
<http://www.icn.ch/>

The International Council of Nurses is a federation of national nurses' associations (NNAs). Founded in 1899, ICN is the world's first and widest reaching international organisation for health professionals, now representing nurses in more than 120 countries. Operated by nurses for nurses, ICN works 'to ensure quality nursing care for all, sound health policies globally, the advancement of nursing knowledge, and the presence worldwide of a respected nursing profession and a competent and satisfied nursing workforce'.

The site enables access to a range of policy and programme areas, press releases and FAQs, as well as fact sheets and guidelines.

National Library of Medicine
<http://www.nlm.nih.gov>

The US National Library of Medicine, the world's largest medical library, maintains a huge and detailed Web site providing a range of resources aimed at both health professionals and patients. Despite the US bias, many of the resources are valuable to a UK audience.

MedlinePlus <http://medlineplus.gov/> is an authoritative and up-to-date source of health information, aimed at both professionals and the general public. It includes links to extensive information from the National Institutes of Health and other trusted sources on over 650 diseases and conditions. It also provides an illustrated medical encyclopedia, a medical dictionary, interactive health tutorials, and the latest health news. The site is updated daily.

Genetics Home Reference <http://ghr.nlm.nih.gov/> is the National Library of Medicine's Web site for consumer information about genetic conditions and the genes or chromosomes responsible for those conditions. *Help Me Understand Genetics* <http://ghr.nlm.nih.gov/info=understandGenetics> presents basic information about genetics in clear language and provides links to other online resources.

Conclusion

The sites included here represent a tiny fraction of the useful information available on the Web, provided by reputable organisations. We hope that having looked at a few Web sites, you will be encouraged to search or browse more widely.

If you are looking for the Web site of a particular organisation, try a Google search (see Chapter 3) – the ranking facility makes it very effective.

Top Tip

GMS contract:
10 key disease areas

CHAPTER **5**

Box 5.1   Chapter objectives

♦ Identify a number of high-quality Web sites on topics relating to specific disease areas.

♦ Give preference to UK sites of interest to nurses in primary care.

♦ Provide a starting point for further exploration.

Introduction

On 1st April 2004, the new General Medical Services (GMS) contract was implemented across the UK, with almost 100% of practices signing up to it. It introduced a quality and outcomes framework, consisting of four domains – clinical standards, organisational standards, additional service standards and patient experience.

This chapter will introduce the reader to a selection of high-quality resources relating to the 10 disease areas contained in the clinical standards domain. Some of these resources were identified using Web sites mentioned in Chapters 3 and 4, for example NMAP (see Chapter 3) and the National electronic Library for Health (NeLH) (see Chapter 4).

For ease of reference and use, this chapter has been presented primarily in the form of tables.

General sources

The resources identified in this section are relevant to several of the disease areas. To avoid repetition, and the attempt to transcribe long URLs, we have listed the parent sites or pages in **Table 5.1**. We encourage readers to visit the sites and browse to find more specific resources.

Visit <http://www.nurseshandbook.co.uk> to find links to all the sites mentioned in this book.

Top Tip

Table 5.1 General sources

Web site	Description
NeLH: National Service Frameworks Zones <http://www.nelh.nhs.uk/nsf/>	NeLH is developing a series of National Service Frameworks (NSFs) Zones, which provide gateways to the key sites and resources related to implementation of the NSFs for all healthcare practitioners and managers. They will include supporting healthcare guidelines and care pathways, and information resources for patients.
	For example: Coronary Heart Disease <http://www.nelh.nhs.uk/nsf/chd/>
NeLH: Specialist Libraries <http://www.nelh.nhs.uk/specialist/>	Also under development. They will contain collections of clinical resources within specialty themes.
	For example: Diabetes <http://libraries.nelh.nhs.uk/diabetes/>
Treatment notes <http://www.nelh.nhs.uk/treatmentnotes/treatmentnotes.asp>	NeLH, National Knowledge Service and Which? Ltd have jointly produced a series of Treatment notes, which offer patients, carers and members of the public access to high-quality health information in a concise easy-to-read format.
	They are in the form of PDF files, including, for example:
	◆ *Breathless due to COPD?*
	◆ *Inhaled Steroids for children with Asthma*
National Institute for Clinical Excellence (NICE) <http://www.nice.org.uk/>	NICE is responsible for providing national guidance on treatments and care for people using the NHS in England and Wales. Their guidance is intended for healthcare professionals, patients and their carers to help them make decisions about treatment and healthcare. The Web site includes sections on guidance, implementation, and how NICE works.

Nurse Prescriber
<http://www.nurse-prescriber.co.uk/>

A free online educational service and information resource 'devoted to all nurse prescribers and healthcare professionals in related fields'. The site includes 'Clinical management plans: a toolkit', which provides examples of CMPs for specific treatments, including diabetes, hypertension and asthma.

PRODIGY Guidance
<http://www.prodigy.nhs.uk/ClinicalGuidance/>

PRODIGY guidance (see Chapter 4) is available for most of these disease areas.

PRODIGY Patient Information
<http://www.prodigy.nhs.uk/PatientInformation/>

Available on various aspects of several disease areas.

Patient UK: Patient support groups
<http://www.patient.co.uk/selfhelp.asp>

Support groups and medical charities have embraced the Internet as a means of providing information, expertise and help; many sites include information aimed at or useful to health professionals.

The Patient UK site includes links to nearly 2000 UK patient support organisations, self-help groups, and health and disease information providers.

Coronary heart disease

Table 5.2   Coronary heart diseases: recommended starting points

Web site	Description
British Heart Foundation <http://www.bhf.org.uk/>	The BHF offers a wide range of literature for patients, but also provides specialist information in the form of Factfiles on relevant treatments or heart conditions.
	For example, BHF Factfile on CHD: <http://www.bhf.org.uk/professionals/index.asp?secondlevel=471>
HealthNet <http://www.healthnet.org.uk/>	A health promotion site, aimed at the public, health professionals and students, developed by the Coronary Prevention Group (an organisation set up by medical experts to promote action on the prevention of CHD). It provides free and accessible information on all aspects of heart disease prevention.
National Heart Forum <http://www.heartforum.org.uk/>	The NHF is an alliance of over 40 national organisations working to reduce the risk of coronary heart disease in the UK. The Web site provides information about their work, policy recommendations and publications.

Stroke and Transient Ischaemic Attacks (TIAs)

Table 5.3   Stroke and Transient Ischaemic Attacks: recommended starting points

Web site	Description
The Stroke Association <http://www.stroke.org.uk/>	The Web site provides a section for professionals at <http://www.stroke.org.uk/professionals/index.html>. It includes information about publications for health professionals, training, community services and research.
Different Strokes <http://www.differentstrokes.co.uk/>	A registered charity providing a unique, free service to younger stroke survivors throughout the United Kingdom. It is 'run by stroke survivors for stroke survivors, for active self help and mutual support'.
US National Institute of Neurological Disorders and Stroke <http://www.ninds.nih.gov/>	Includes a detailed online guide called 'Stroke: Hope Through Research' <http://www.ninds.nih.gov/health_and_medical/pubs/stroke_hope_through_research.htm>. Particular attention is given to risk factors.

Hypertension

Table 5.4: Hypertension: recommended starting points

Web site	Description
The British Hypertension Society <http://www.hyp.ac.uk/bhs/default.htm>	Provides a medical and scientific research forum 'to enable sharing of cutting edge research in order to understand the origin of high blood pressure and improve its treatment.' 'Factfiles for Health Professionals' are listed at: <http://www.hyp.ac.uk/bhs/publications_leaflets.htm>.
Blood Pressure Association <http://www.bpassoc.org.uk/>	A British charity, launched in October 2000, which aims to support health professionals by developing 'a range of information materials that are short, simple and practical'; some are available to download and others can be ordered via the site. The site also provides information on medication, lifestyle, and general issues related to high blood pressure.
'Your Guide to Lowering High Blood Pressure' <http://www.nhlbi.nih.gov/hbp/index.html>	A site intended for people who are interested in learning more about preventing and controlling high blood pressure. Based on US National Heart, Lung, and Blood Institute clinical guidelines and research studies, it provides up-to-date practical information on high blood pressure.

Hypothyroidism

Table 5.5: Hypothyroidism: recommended starting points

Web site	Description
The British Thyroid Foundation <http://www.btf-thyroid.org/>	A patient-led charity dedicated to helping those with thyroid disorders. Their Web site includes information about thyroid function and disorders, with sections aimed at patients and at health professionals.
British Society for Paediatric Endocrinology and Diabetes <http://www.bsped.org.uk/index.html>	A page of notes on Hypothyroidism in Childhood is available at <http://www.bsped.org.uk/patients/nick/HYPOTHY.htm>. This is part of a series of structured A4 hand-outs designed for parent & patient use that can be printed off or downloaded for modification locally by professionals.
MayoClinic.com: Hyperthyroidism page <http://www.mayoclinic.com/invoke.cfm?id=DS00344>	This site aims to 'empower people to manage their health' by providing up-to-date health information produced by medical experts.

Diabetes

Table 5.6: Diabetes: recommended starting points

Web site	Description
Royal College of General Practitioners <http://www.rcgp.org.uk/>	The National Collaborating Centre for Primary Care (commissioned by NICE) has developed guidelines which can be found at <http://www.rcgp.org.uk/nccpc/completedguidelines.asp?menuid=83>.
Diabetes UK <http://www.diabetes.org.uk>	The site contains information on Diabetes UK (formerly the British Diabetics Association), its services and publications, and includes a section for healthcare professionals.
Juvenile Diabetes Research Foundation <http://www.jdrf.org.uk>	A section for health professionals provides information on progress, research and treatment for diabetes.

Mental health

Table 5.7: Mental health: recommended starting points

Web site	Description
Mind <http://www.mind.org.uk/>	The Web site of the 'leading mental health charity in England and Wales' covers its works and policies, and includes a range of clear and detailed fact sheets and booklets.
Mental Health Foundation <http://www.mentalhealth.org.uk/>	A comprehensive source of information about mental health issues and the work of the Foundation, as well as a gateway to some of the other resources on mental health, both in the UK and overseas.
WHO Guide to Mental and Neurological Health in Primary Care: A Guide to Mental and Neurological Ill Health in Adults, Children and Adolescents <http://www.mentalneurologicalprimarycare.org/>	This guide is intended 'to support primary care professionals, primary care organisations and local user groups in their delivery of primary care mental and neurological health services. It deals with conditions frequently seen in primary care, or those that have a high profile, and which can be managed effectively by general practitioners (GPs) and their teams, supported as appropriate by secondary care.

Chronic obstructive pulmonary disease (COPD)

Table 5.8: Chronic obstructive pulmonary disease (COPD): recommended starting points

Web site	Description
BestTreatments: COPD <http://www.besttreatments.co.uk/btuk/conditions/14421.html>	Part of a site developed by the BMJ publishing group, looking at the effectiveness of treatments for chronic conditions, covering treatments, symptoms, diagnosis and progression of the condition.
British Lung Foundation <http://www.lunguk.org/>	The BLF provides information on all aspects of lung conditions. A page on COPD can be found at <http://www.lunguk.org/copdasp?dis=13>. Information about the support network, the Breathe Easy Club, is at <http://www.lunguk.org/support-groups.asp>.
Netdoctor: Chronic Bronchitis <http://www.netdoctor.co.uk/diseases/facts/smokerslung.htm>	An article on the NetDoctor site on Chronic bronchitis, emphysema and COPD ('smoker's lung') provides a brief, clear overview of symptoms, causes and treatment, including lifestyle changes.

Asthma

Table 5.9: **Asthma: recommended starting points**

Web site	Description
Asthma UK (formerly the National Asthma Campaign) <http://www.asthma.org.uk/>	The site provides a range of clearly presented information about asthma, and includes a section for health professionals. Patient information leaflets are available in at least 16 languages to help healthcare professionals working with patients whose first language is not English.
BTS/SIGN British Guideline on the management of Asthma <http://www.brit-thoracic.org.uk/sign/index.htm>	The clinical guideline was produced by the British Thoracic Society (the official body of medical professionals with an interest in respiratory disease) and the Scottish Intercollegiate Guidelines Network in 2003, and updated in 2004. The site also includes patient information, posters and interactive case histories.
US National, Heart, Blood and Lung Institute <http://www.nhlbi.nih.gov/>	A number of fact sheets are available at: <http://www.nhlbi.nih.gov/health/public/lung/index.htm>

Epilepsy

Table 5.10: Epilepsy: recommended starting points

Web site	Description
National Society for Epilepsy <http://www.epilepsynse.org.uk> e-epilepsy <http://www.e-epilepsy.org.uk/>	The NSE site provides a range of information on epilepsy, treatment and many aspects of living with epilepsy. Their e-epilepsy site is aimed at health professionals, and includes a library of articles, literature reviews, news coverage, drug information and a professional enquiry service, with the facility to browse through responses to previous enquiries.
Epilepsy Action (British Epilepsy Association) <http://www.epilepsy.org.uk/>	The 'largest member-led epilepsy organisation in Britain', providing support and information for people with epilepsy, their families, carers and friends. The Web site provides information about epilepsy, drug treatments and research news, and includes special sections for teenagers and younger children.
US National Institute of Neurological Disorders and Stroke <http://www.ninds.nih.gov/>	NINDS has produced a web page called 'Seizures and Epilepsy: hope through research'. It includes detailed information about causes, diagnosis, prevention and treatment of epilepsy. <http://www.ninds.nih.gov/health_and_medical/pubs/seizures_and_epilepsy_htr.htm>

Cancer

Table 5.11: Cancer: recommended starting points

Web site	Description
Cancer charities – examples	
◆ Cancer Bacup <http://www.cancerbacup.org.uk/Home>	There are several general nationwide cancer charities in the UK, as well as a range of organisations concerned with specific types of cancer. Most of the larger groups have an impressive Web presence.
◆ Cancer Research UK <http://www.cancerresearchuk.org/>	
◆ Macmillan Cancer Relief <http://www.macmillan.org.uk/>	
◆ Marie Curie Cancer Care <http://www.mariecurie.org.uk/>	
NHSIA Cancer Information Services <http://www.nhsia.nhs.uk/cancer/pages/>	A collection of Cancer data intended to improve the care of cancer patients in England, driven by the implementation of national and local initiatives for recording, using and analysing good quality information.
CancerNet <http://cancernet.nci.nih.gov/>	Produced by the US National Cancer Institute; provides detailed information on a range of cancers, including symptoms, treatment and follow-up care.

Conclusion

In researching this chapter, our difficulty was not in identifying high-quality sites, but in selecting just a few for each disease area. This selection should be regarded as introductory, and by no means exhaustive: space constraints forced us to exclude far more sites than we could include. We hope that as you become more experienced as Internet users, and more familiar with the search tools and medical sites discussed in earlier chapters, you will be able to identify relevant high-quality sites on these and other disease areas for yourself.

Childhood immunisation

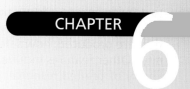

CHAPTER

6

Box 6.1 Chapter objectives

♦ Identify a selection of high-quality Web sites relevant to childhood vaccination.

♦ Introduce the reader to some more general sources on vaccines and medicines.

♦ Give preference to UK sites of interest to nurses in primary care.

Introduction

In this chapter, we have identified sites covering topics such as: immunisation schedules; vaccine-preventable diseases; how vaccination leads to immunity; types of vaccine; production and safety. As well as sites focussing on childhood immunisation, we cover some sources providing general information on vaccination, vaccines and medicines.

UK Government sites

Immunisation Against Infectious Disease – 'The Green Book'

<http://www.dh.gov.uk/PolicyAndGuidance/HealthAndSocialCareTopics/Green Book/fs/en>

The Green Book is the Department of Health's (DH) recommendations regarding vaccination in the UK. A number of bodies contribute to the writing of the Green Book, including the DH and the Health Protection Agency. The recommendations are based on those made by the Joint Committee of Vaccination and Immunisation (JCVI). Individual chapters are updated or introduced to correspond with new developments or changes to the vaccination schedule. As new chapters are written or existing chapters are updated, they are posted on the DH Web site which should be checked regularly to ensure the most current guidelines are being followed.

NHS Immunisation information

<http://www.immunisation.org.uk>

This is the official Department of Health Web site on immunisation, providing 'comprehensive, up-to-date and accurate' information on vaccines and immunisation. It provides the full immunisation schedule (**Figure 6.1**), which is structured to provide links to information about diseases and vaccines. A detailed section of the site called 'About immunisation' covers topics such as how vaccines work, how they are produced, how safety is monitored, and what is meant by 'herd immunity'. Other features include FAQs, news stories, links to useful Web sites, and a library of printed resources available to view, download or to order from the Department of Health for both healthcare professionals and parents. A selection of these leaflets is available in several different languages.

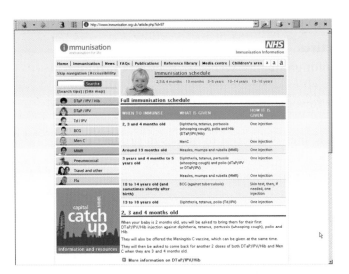

Figure 6.1 *NHS Immunisation Information – immunisation schedule*

MMR The facts

<http://www.mmrthefacts.nhs.uk/>

This site is also compiled by the Immunisation Information team at the DH. It makes available a range of materials designed to provide both parents and health professionals with the latest information on MMR (the combined vaccine against measles, mumps and rubella). A section called 'MMR Library' lists key research, along with a glossary and a section on 'What the experts say'. A range of fact sheets (in 10 languages) is available in PDF format.

UK professional guides

Childhood immunisation: a guide for healthcare professionals

<http://www.bma.org.uk/ap.nsf/Content/immunisation>

This is a report by the British Medical Association, Board of Science and Education, published in June 2003, which reviews the principles of vaccination and immunisation in the UK in children aged 0–5 years. Vaccines not included in the UK immunisation programme, but given to children if clinically indicated, are also mentioned. The report is available in PDF format.

Childhood vaccination factfile

<http://www.rcn.org.uk/publications/pdf/ChildhoodVaccinationFactfile.pdf>

Written by key healthcare professionals from the Royal College of Nursing (RCN) and the Community Practitioners and Health Visitors Association (CPHVA), this information pack was produced with the aim of 'providing healthcare professionals with accurate information, covering all key aspects of the immunisation of children'. The document is available in PDF format, requiring Adobe Acrobat Reader.

UK vaccine industry sites

Sanofi Pasteur MSD Ltd

<http://www.spmsd.co.uk/>

Provided by Sanofi Pasteur MSD Ltd, this site supports their aim of 'increasing the understanding of the value of vaccines and vaccination by providing relevant and accurate information on their quality, safety and efficacy.' The public area of the site provides information about diseases and about childhood, adult and travel vaccines. Healthcare professionals can register (using their GMC/NMC/RPS number) for access to a password-protected area of the site where access to VIS Online is also available. VIS Online is designed for healthcare professionals 'seeking advice on individual clinical queries/problems relating to vaccination'.

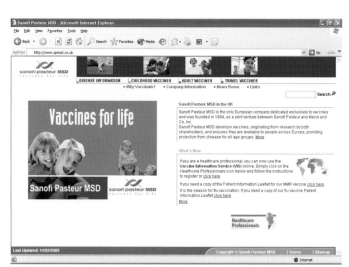

Figure 6.2   *Sanofi Pasteur MSD Ltd*

UK Vaccine Industry Group

<http://www.uvig.org/>

The UK Vaccine Industry Group, working within the Association of the British Pharmaceutical Industry (ABPI), 'aims to promote the positive benefits of vaccination as a key element in improving the health of the nation' and 'to represent the UK vaccine industry to all interested parties'. The main feature of the site is a series of factsheets, available as Web pages or PDF files, covering topics such as production and safety of vaccines, childhood immunisation and travel vaccines.

UK medicines

British National Formulary (BNF) Online

<http://www.bnf.org>

The BNF (**Figure 6.3**) is a joint publication of the British Medical Association and the Royal Pharmaceutical Society of Great Britain. It aims to provide pre-scribers, pharmacists and other healthcare professionals with 'key informa-tion on the selection, prescribing, dispensing and administration of medicines'. The Web site is intended 'to support healthcare professionals familiar with the scope and organisation of information within the BNF and as such assumes the level of professional training required to appropriately interpret the advice contained herein'. Access is free but registration is required.

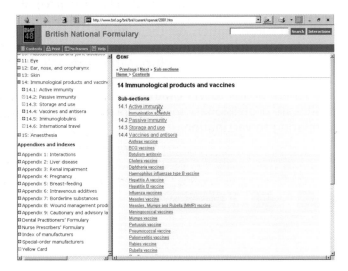

Figure 6.3   *BNF – Section 14: Immunological products and vaccines*

electronic Medicines Compendium

<http://www.medicines.org.uk/emc.aspx>

The electronic Medicines Compendium provides free access to current and comprehensive information on prescription and over-the-counter medicines available in the UK. Information has been provided by the pharmaceutical industry and for each medicine includes the Summary of Product Characteristics (SPC) and, in some cases, the Patient Information Leaflet (PIL).

International sites

MedlinePlus: Childhood Immunisation

<http://www.nlm.nih.gov/medlineplus/childhoodimmunization.html>

This page provides an extensive list of links to authoritative sources of information on a wide range of related topics. Despite the US bias, it is particularly useful for information on understanding how vaccinations work.

Quackwatch: Misconceptions about immunisation
<http://www.quackwatch.org/03HealthPromotion/immu/immu00.html>

Quackwatch, Inc. is a not-for-profit corporation whose purpose is 'to combat health-related frauds, myths, fads, and fallacies'. This page dispels at least 10 common misconceptions about immunisation, and provides links to reliable information sources.

Conclusion

The sites selected for this chapter are only a selection of the vaccine-related Web sites on the Internet. There are also a great many useful, authoritative Web sites relating to single diseases. (For example, the Web site of the Meningitis Trust <http://www.meningitis-trust.org/> provides clearly presented information about the disease, as well as about treatment and vaccination.) Using the sites we have identified in earlier chapters, and the search skills you have acquired, we hope that you will be equipped to identify other sources for yourself.

Travel health

CHAPTER 7

Box 7.1   Chapter objectives

♦ Identify a selection of high-quality Web sites relevant to travel health.
♦ Introduce the reader to international sites as well as UK sites.

Introduction

Every year, residents of the United Kingdom go on more than 63.5 million overseas journeys. Now that international travel is commonplace, there is a frequent need for authoritative, reliable, up-to-date information on travel health. In this chapter, we have identified a range of sites covering topics such as vaccination, diseases, outbreaks and other information for travellers, as well as sites aimed primarily at health professionals.

For general sites on vaccination, vaccines and medicines, such as VIS Online (**see Figure 7.1**) and the British National Formulary (BNF Online), please refer to Chapter 6.

UK Government sites

The National Travel Health Network and Centre (NaTHNaC)
<http://www.nathnac.org/>

Funded by the Department of Health (DH), NaTHNaC has been created to promote clinical standards in travel medicine with the goal of 'protecting the health of the British traveller'. The site is divided into two sections: 'For Health Professionals' (**Figure 7.2**) and 'For Travellers'. The Professionals' area includes Health Risk Information Sheets, which provide general health information on infectious and non-infectious health risks that travellers may encounter whilst overseas. Information, which may result in a change in travel health advice or practice, is posted in a section called 'Clinical updates.'

Health advice for travellers
<http://www.dh.gov.uk/PolicyAndGuidance/HealthAdviceForTravellers/fs/en>

This area of the Department of Health Web site contains advice for travellers about 'planning ahead, staying healthy and getting treatment elsewhere in the world'. It

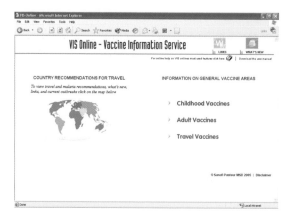

Figure 7.1   *VIS Online*

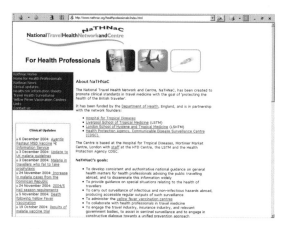

Figure 7.2   *NaTHNaC –*
Health Professionals' section

also provides information on how to access free reduced-cost emergency care in most other European countries. A section on 'Latest health updates' provides regularly updated alerts on outbreaks all over the world together with advice for travellers about staying safe.

Foreign and Commonwealth Office

<http://www.fco.gov.uk/travel>

The FCO Travel Advice Web site is designed to help British travellers to make informed decisions about travelling abroad. It includes official FCO Travel Advice notices for over 200 countries 'based on the most accurate and up-to-date information available'. The Travel Health section provides information about diseases, injuries and precautions. Other areas of the site cover insurance, passports, money and consular assistance.

Health Information for Overseas Travel (The 'Yellow Book', 2001)

<http://www.archive.official-documents.co.uk/document/doh/hinfo/index.htm>

This handbook was first issued in 1995 and updated in 2001; it is of particular value to doctors and practice nurses giving travel health advice in primary care, and is now commonly referred to as the UK 'Yellow Book'. It starts with descriptions (by continental group) of the disease and health risks most likely to be encountered by travellers, with recommendations for their prevention; later chapters include advice about accident and injury prevention, food and water hygiene, protection against insect bites, environmental hazards and sexual health.

HPA Malaria Reference Laboratory (MRL)
<http://www.lshtm.ac.uk/pmbu/PHLS/>

The Malaria Reference Laboratory (MRL) of the Health Protection Agency (formerly PHLS) provides 'an integrated service for public health in relation to malaria'. The site provides contact details for their Advisory Service, as well as a link to Malaria Prevention Guidelines provided by the HPA at <http://www.hpa.org.uk/infections/topics_az/malaria/guidelines.htm>.

TRAVAX
<http://www.travax.scot.nhs.uk/>

The Travel Medicine Division at Health Protection Scotland produce TRAVAX, 'an interactive online database providing up to the minute travel health information', which is provided as a NHS resource for healthcare professionals who advise patients about avoiding illness when travelling abroad. It is available only to registered users: it is free of charge for all using the service for NHS purposes in Scotland; there is a charge for NHS users in other parts of the United Kingdom.

UK Industry Sites

VIS Online

<http://www.spmsd.co.uk/>

VIS Online is supplied by Sanofi Pasteur MSD. It is an easy to use, free source of information for healthcare professionals. It is updated every working day and provides reliable information on travel issues, country recommendations, malaria and outbreaks. It also gives comprehensive information on the full range of their vaccines, whether for children, adults or for travel, in a simple A–Z format. The 'What's new' section will also keep you up-to-date on vaccine-related issues.

International Sites

World Health Organization (WHO): International Travel and Health
<http://www.who.int/ith/>

These pages are addressed primarily to medical and public health professionals who provide health advice to travellers, and are intended 'to give guidance on the full range of significant health issues associated with travel'. Where possible information is presented in a form 'readily accessible to interested travellers and non-medical readers'.

CDC Travelers' Health
<http://www.cdc.gov/travel/>

The Centers for Disease Control and Prevention (CDC) is an agency of the US Department of Health and Human Services, and is the leading Federal Agency for protecting the health and safety of people at home and abroad. The site provides a detailed collection of official information on travel health, including sections on destinations, outbreaks, diseases and vaccinations.

It also includes the full text of *Health Information for International Travel 2003–2004* — the 'Yellow Book' <http://www.cdc.gov/travel/yb/index.htm>, which is published every two years by CDC as a reference for those who advise international travellers of health risks. The Yellow Book is written primarily for healthcare providers.

World Health Organization (WHO): Communicable Disease Surveillance and Response
<http://www.who.int/csr/en/>

CSR is the division of WHO concerned with the surveillance, prevention and control of communicable diseases, including newly emerging or re-emerging infections. The site includes Disease Outbreak News at <http://www.who.int/csr/don/en/> and a freely accessible electronic edition of the Weekly Epidemiological Record <http://www.who.int/wer/en/>, as well as information on a variety of infectious diseases.

International Association for Medical Assistance to Travellers
<http://www.iamat.org>

IAMAT is a non-profit organisation established in 1960. Their aim is 'to advise travellers about health risks, the geographical distribution of diseases worldwide and immunisation requirements for all countries.' Publications available on the site include the World Immunization Chart <http://www.iamat.org/pdf/WorldImmunization.pdf> and World Malaria Risk Chart <http://www.iamat.org/pdf/WorldMalariaRisk.pdf>, both in **PDF** format, therefore requiring **Adobe Acrobat Reader** to view them

Medline Plus Traveler's Health
<http://www.nlm.nih.gov/medlineplus/travelershealth.html>

This site provides access to a detailed and varied compendium of authoritative resources on a range of issues related to travel.

Other useful sites

Try looking up the Health Protection Agency or the BBC travel health page by typing them in to Google.

Conclusion

As with earlier chapters, this should be regarded as an introductory selection, not an exhaustive list. However, we have given preference to major sites providing authoritative content, all of which are good examples of the use of the Internet to improve travel health knowledge and increase awareness of health risks.

Advanced searching

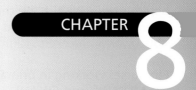

CHAPTER

8

Box 8.1 – Chapter objectives

♦ Highlight the need to be aware of a range of tools when searching the Internet for research-based nursing and medical information.

♦ Provide a practical guide on how to search MEDLINE and CINAHL.

♦ Provide a practical guide to searching two key medical/scientific search engines – Google Scholar and Scirus.

♦ Demonstrate, through worked examples, how you can use these tools to find information specific to your needs.

Introduction

Although the search services discussed in Chapter 3 provide an excellent means of finding information on the Internet, there are times when more sophisticated search tools are required, especially when you are looking for peer-reviewed, research-based information. Typically, such information is stored in indexing and abstracting databases, such as MEDLINE and CINAHL.

This chapter, therefore, provides a *practical* guide to help you search these (and other) resources. Using these tools, nurses working in primary care can readily access current research and see what the state of knowledge is – referred to as the evidence-base – in any given topic.

In addition to providing an analysis of the traditional medical/nursing databases, attention will also be given to a number of *new* medical search engines, such as Google Scholar and Scirus.

Top Tip

All the resources discussed in this chapter are either freely available, or are available free of charge to NHS professionals via the National Library for Health <http://www.library.nhs.uk/>. If in doubt, ask you local NHS or University Librarian.

Databases

There are many databases health professionals can turn to when trying to determine the research that has been published on a given topic. A researcher interested in clinical trials would appreciate the wealth of information available through the Clinical Trials database <http://www.clinicaltrials.gov/> a US-based site, whilst a psychiatrist interested in, say, the phenomenon of Internet addiction would find the Psychological Abstracts database <http://www.apa.org/psycinfo/> a rich source of data.

For nurses working in primary care, however, the two most useful databases are MEDLINE and CINAHL.

MEDLINE

Address: <http://www.ncbi.nlm.nih.gov/PubMed>

Access restrictions None – freely available

MEDLINE, produced by US National Library of Medicine, is the world's premier biomedical database. Dating from 1966 (although the printed version, Index Medicus, dates from 1879) the MEDLINE database currently contains over 11 million bibliographic references and abstracts drawn from more than 4300 biomedical journals.

Searching MEDLINE

Although MEDLINE uses a highly structured vocabulary – MeSH – it is nevertheless possible to search for articles using common terms and phrases. For example, the search 'managing pressure sores' identifies a number of potentially useful articles, from journals such as *Nursing Management*, and the *British Journal of Nursing* (**Figure 8.1**).

Type in your search criteria here – it could be a topic or an author's name, then click on the 'Go' button on the right

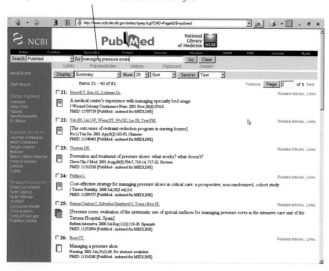

Figure 8.1 *Results from a simple MEDLINE search – not all articles are from English-language journals*

While these particular articles would prove useful, a quick glance at the results page (**Figure 8.1**) shows that others may be less so. Unless you speak Chinese, the second reference listed would be inaccessible, whilst those that focused on highly specific aspects of pressure sore management – such as comparing silicone and polymer dressings – may be irrelevant.

To counter such problems a more sophisticated approach to searching is required. **Box 8.2** provides a worked example as to how a MEDLINE search can be constructed so that *only* highly relevant articles are identified.

Box 8.2 – Advanced MEDLINE searching

Question

Is there any up-to-date research – published in nursing journals within the past two years – that considers the role of diet in the prevention and management of coronary heart disease?

Answer & Methodology.

1. Log-on to the MEDLINE database <http://www.ncbi.nlm.nih.gov/PubMed>.
2. In the **Search** box, enter the term *diet* – click the **Go** button.

A list of citations that contain the term 'diet' are displayed – 20 references at a time.

3. Next, use the **Clear** button to empty the search box and then enter the phrase *coronary heart disease*. Click the Go button.

Two separate sets of results have now been created. Set 1 contains articles about diet, whilst Set 2 has articles relating to coronary heart disease. These sets now need to be combined using the AND Boolean operator.

4. Click on the **History** button to see your search history.

Here you will see two sets – one for each subject we have searched for – along with the number of articles MEDLINE has retrieved.

5. Use the **Clear** button to empty the search box and enter the set numbers you want to combine. When combining search sets always prefix the set number with the # character. Boolean search operators, AND, OR, and NOT **must** be entered in upper case.

In this example we enter:

#1 AND #2

Press **Go**

As this search produced over 6000 references, various limits can be applied to focus the search to the more pertinent articles.

6. Click on the **Limits** option (**Figure 8.2**).

Use the **Entrez Date** option to limit the results to articles published in the past 2 years.

Use the **Language** option to limit the results to articles that are in English.

Use the **Subsets** option to limit the results articles that are in nursing journals.

Press **Go**.

Comment

This example shows the benefit of using the advanced search facilities available within MEDLINE. With just a few clicks an unmanageable number of articles (6221) was reduced to just 14.

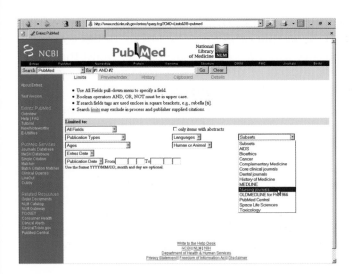

Figure 8.2 *Using the 'Limits' menu in MEDLINE*

Further help

For further information and help on how to search MEDLINE effectively see the MEDLINE Training manuals at: <http://www.nlm.nih.gov/bsd/pubmed _tutorial/m1001.html>.

CINAHL

Address:	1. NHS access: <http://nhs.dialog.com/>
	2. HE access: <http://gateway.uk.ovid.com>
	3. Public access: <http://www.cinahl.com/>
Access restrictions	1. Only available via a computer connected to the NHSnet, or to eligible users with an **Athens** username and password.
	2. Only available via a computer connected to the JANET network, or to eligible users with an **Athens** username and password.
	3. Available to all. Annual membership: $20.00

CINAHL – the Cumulative Index to Nursing and Allied Health Literature – can be seen as the nursing equivalent to MEDLINE. As of November 2004 the database holds more than 1,000,000 records, derived from over 1700 nursing, allied health and consumer health journals.

Searching CINAHL

Although the CINAHL database can be searched by simply entering any search term or phrase, it is also possible to search the database using CINAHL subject headings. One of the advantages of using a controlled vocabulary is that like resources are grouped together, irrespective of the specific terms individual authors may have used in their work. For example, one author may use the term 'baldness' whilst another may use 'alopecia' to describe the same condition. CINAHL subject headings overcome the problem of synonyms by forcing indexers to use a set of preferred terms. As a consequence, subject-heading searching is far more precise than simple free-text searching.

Box 8.3 provides a worked example showing how a CINAHL search can be constructed using CINAHL subject headings.

Other databases

In addition to the databases described here there are many other subject-specific databases accessible via the Internet. Brief details of these are provided in **Table 8.1**.

Medical search engines

The traditional Internet search services like Google (see Chapter 3) are not particularly useful when trying to identify high-quality, peer-reviewed research papers. For example, although a Google search for 'stroke' *will* identify useful sites – such as the National Stroke Association – it will also find web pages that advise you on how to improve your swimming *stroke*, or modify your two-*stroke* motorcycle engine!

Even more problematic is the fact that much of the high-quality content published in scientific journals cannot be indexed by the usual search tools, as access is restricted to paying subscribers.

Box 8.3 – Advanced CINAHL searching

Question

Is there any research that considers both the epidemiology and the prevention of shingles?

Answer & Methodology

1. Log-on to the CINAHL database. In this example, I will use the OVID service, available to HE institutions <http://gateway.uk.ovid.com/>.

2. In the search box enter Shingles and hit the Search button.

As Shingles is not recognised as a CINAHL subject heading, the search is mapped to the most appropriate heading, Herpes Zoster.

3. Click on the **Continue** button.

The resulting display shows all the topical subheadings that can be applied to this term. These include complications, drug therapy and prevention and control.

4. Select the subheadings relevant to this search – **prevention and control** and **epidemiology**. Hit the **Continue** button.

5. The search is executed and the only articles that are retrieved are those that focus on the epidemiology and prevention of shingles. In this example, just 66 citations were identified. If this was still felt to be too many, the search could be further refined using the **Limits** menu.

Comment

This search successfully highlights the effectiveness of using CINAHL subject headings and topical subheadings when you want to undertake a comprehensive search. All relevant articles – whether they contain the word shingles or the more technical term, herpes zoster – are successfully retrieved in one search set.

Table 8.1   Other research databases: a quick reference guide

Database:	AMED
Address	<http://www.library.nhs.uk/>
Access	Available to NHS staff – via NLH
Analysis	The AMED database focuses on the disciplines of complementary and allied medicine.
Database:	British Nursing Index
Address	<http://www.library.nhs.uk/>
Access	Available to NHS staff – via NLH
Analysis	Describing itself as the 'premier database for the support of education, research, practice and development of UK nurses, midwives, health visitors, and related staff', the British Nursing Index (BNI) is a tightly-focused, bibliographic database comprising over 250 of the most popular and important journal sources in the nursing and midwifery fields.
Database:	Clinical Trials Database
Address	<http://www.clinicaltrials.gov>
Access	Free
Analysis	The Clinical Trials database aims to 'link patients to medical research'. Each trial in the database contains a description highlighting its purpose, what phase it has reached, and whether or not new recruits are still being accepted.
Database:	Cochrane Database of Systematic Reviews
Address	<http://www.nelh.nhs.uk/cochrane.asp>
Access	Free to all UK residents
Analysis	The Cochrane Database contains a series of original reviews that attempt to determine whether treatments for specific and identified conditions are effective. Conclusions are reached by looking at all the research that has been published on a defined topic. Recognising that some pieces of research are more authoritative than others, the authors of the Cochrane Reviews focus on research that was conducted using the randomised controlled trials (RCT's) methodology. Studies conducted using RCT's are less prone to bias and produce more reliable conclusions.
Database:	PsycINFO
Address	<http://www.library.nhs.uk/>
Access	Available to NHS staff – via NLH
Analysis	Produced by the American Psychological Association, the PsycINFO database provides extensive international coverage of the literature on psychology and allied fields.

In recognition of these problems, a new breed of Internet search services – aimed at the research and scholarly communities – has been developed. Two of the most useful are Google Scholar and Scirus.

Google Scholar

Address:	<http://scholar.google.com/>
Access restrictions	None – freely available. *Note: Access to some full-text access may be limited to online subscribers.*

Over the past few years developers at Google have worked with a number of key scientific and medical publishers to gain access to material that would not usually be accessible to indexing services. This information has been brought together and is now accessible via Google Scholar.

Searching Google Scholar is as easy as searching Google (see Chapter 3). For example, a search for 'preventing falls in the elderly' (**Figure 8.3**) identifies a range of useful research papers from sources such as the Cochrane Library, *BMJ* and the *New England Journal of Medicine*. More significantly, papers with the most citations (which therefore tend to be the most important papers) are ranked highest.

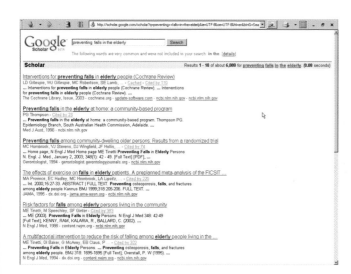

Figure 8.3 *Simple search using Google Scholar*

Although it is not *always* possible to link from the citation to the full-text of an article, as this service includes resources held at HighWire (which at the time of writing provides free access to around 800,000 free full-text articles), many articles can be accessed free of charge.

Google Scholar, however, has not been permitted to index research papers published by Elsevier, the world's largest scientific publisher. To access these you need to use the Scirus search service.

Scirus

Address:	<http://www.scirus.com/>
Access restrictions	None – freely available. *Note: Access to some full-text articles may be limited to online subscribers.*

Developed by Elsevier Science, the Scirus search engine focuses exclusively on Web sites with scientific content. Web pages on topics *other* than science are excluded from the Scirus database of 167 million pages.

As with Google Scholar, Scirus does not restrict its searching to Web sites. This search engine also indexes the contents of more than 1800 full-text journal articles – drawn principally from Elsevier's impressive stable of scientific and medical publications – plus the contents of databases, such as MEDLINE. Thus, through a single interface, users have access to some of the best scientific pages on the Web *and* direct access to 5.5 million online articles.

By providing a one-stop search service, Scirus strives to disclose as much scientific information as possible, even if some of this information is not freely available.

An example of how the Scirus search engine was used to answer a specific question is provided in **Box 8.4**.

Box 8.4 – Searching Scirus

Question

Is there any scholarly research that considers the effectiveness of ginger in managing nausea?

Answer & Methodology

One of the problems when searching the Internet for information about alternative therapies is that they typically identify numerous hits, many of which have no scientific basis. By using the Scirus search tool, searches can be limited to scientific Web sites and articles published in the peer-reviewed literature.

1. Log on to Scirus <http://www.scirus.com/>. As in this example we wish to combine two concepts – the advanced search option is selected.

2. In the first search box, key-in *nausea*. In the second box, enter the term *ginger*. As we wish to combine both concepts the default **AND** Boolean operator is selected. Hit the **Search** button.

3. From the results page there is an opportunity to look at scientific Web sites that are relevant to this question, resources from journal articles, or both.

4. From the Web results page there are links to around 4000 sites (**Figure 8.4**), including resources developed by the American Academy of Family Physicians <http://www.aafp.org/afp/20011115/tips/4.html> and the University of Oxford <http://www.jr2.ox.ac.uk/bandolier/booth/alternat/AT128.html>.

5. From the Journal articles results page, some 238 papers are identified, including articles in *Obstetrics and Gynaecology and the Journal of Family Practice*.

Comment

The Scirus search service enables you to find both high-quality Web sites *and* peer-reviewed articles through a single interface.

Use Boolean operators to get more specific results

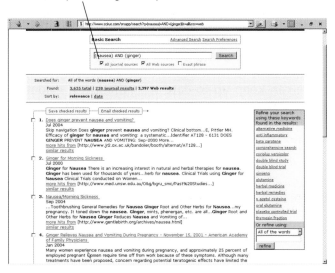

Figure 8.4 *Search results from Scirus*

Databases or medical search engines – a comparison

This chapter has highlighted two approaches – bibliographic databases and medical search engines – to finding high-quality, peer-reviewed information on the Internet. The question begs, therefore, which is the best? Inevitably the answer to this question depends on what you are looking for.

Table 8.2 provides a summary of the strengths and weaknesses of each approach. Using this table you can decide which approach best meets your needs.

Table 8.2 Databases or medical search engines – a comparison

Approach	Strengths	Weaknesses
Databases	◆ Use of 'limit' features – to restrict article to English or those that are published in nursing journals – means that you do not have to sift though irrelevant papers. ◆ Use of subject headings means that highly precise and focused searches can be undertaken.	◆ Can be more difficult to use. ◆ The search is limited to research papers – Web sites tend be excluded.
Medical search services	◆ Easy to use. ◆ A broad range of resources (research papers and Web sites) is indexed.	◆ It is more difficult to construct a highly precise search. ◆ Although the Web sites identified will be scientific in nature, these will not have been peer-reviewed, so their accuracy cannot be assured.

Conclusion

The wealth of resources available via these research databases and medical search services is staggering. Indeed, the MEDLINE database alone indexes over 400,000 new articles every year. Being aware of these resources and, more importantly, having the skills to interrogate them effectively, ensures that nurses in primary care can keep up-to-date with the latest evidence-based research.

Quality of health information on the Internet

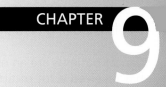

CHAPTER **9**

Box 9.1 Chapter objectives

♦ Highlight a number of the more dubious health claims that are perpetrated on the Internet.

♦ Discuss a number of initiatives that have been developed to help counter the problem of medical misinformation.

♦ Provide tips and advice to help you evaluate the information you find.

Introduction

As we saw at the end of Chapter 3, the quality of health information on the Internet is extremely variable. In this chapter we investigate this concept further, discuss what attempts are being made to regulate health information on the Internet and, most importantly, provide practical guidelines that will help you appraise the quality of the information you find.

Misinformation on the Web

Although examples of medical misinformation on the Internet are numerous, analysis shows that they all fit within one of the following distinct groups:

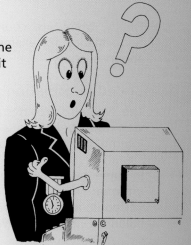

♦ **'Cure-all' remedies and lifestyle scams**
Here a single alternative therapy is presented as a 'magic bullet' solution.

♦ **Biased information**
Only one side of the argument is presented to the reader.

♦ **Dangerous devices**
Sites in this category typically try to sell the unwary consumer a medical device that should only be used by a qualified professional.

We will look in turn at each of these categories, giving examples of these forms of misinformation. Using the searching skills you learned in Chapter 3, you will be able to find many of these sites for yourself.

'Cure-all' remedies and lifestyle scams

It should come as no surprise to learn that the Internet is used to peddle various miracle cures and lifestyle-enhancing drugs. The cost of setting up a credible looking Web site is negligible, whilst the potential profits are huge.

Cancer patients are an obvious target group and one 'cure-all' treatment that has received a lot of attention over the past couple of years is laetrile (also known as 'vitamin B17'), a concoction made of apricot seeds. If you already have cancer you are advised to start eating apricot seeds, safe in the knowledge that this will lead to a cure.

What such sites fail to disclose are the results of the clinical trials that have taken place into laetrile. These show that laetrile has no anticancer activity in humans, and that the side-effects of this 'therapy' mirror the symptoms of cyanide poisoning. (For further details see <http://cancernet.nci.nih.gov/cancertopics/pdq/cam/laetrile>.)

> *If something sounds too good to be true – it probably is.*

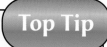
Top Tip

Medical quackery is a business that sells false hope. Not all of this business, however, is aimed at the chronically ill. Many sites prey on the wishful thinking of those who seek shortcuts to weight loss and improvements in their personal appearance and performance. For example, there are sites offering slimming soaps that help you lose weight while you shower, or shampoos that can cure baldness.

Finally, there are countless sites that promise to improve your sexual performance, for example by selling you a 'male skin patch' that claims to enhance virility.

Biased information

The Web also provides a vehicle for every pressure group to promote their views and beliefs to a worldwide audience. Consequently, another issue Internet users need to be alert to is biased information.

In some cases this may be easy to spot (and avoid). Anyone looking for information on, say, the effectiveness of the morning-after pill (mifepristone) will appreciate that they are unlikely to find an objective and balanced view at the Web sites of pro-life organisations.

In some cases, however, bias can be far more subtle and harder to detect. For example there are sites that present, in a highly persuasive way, the arguments against vaccination. Although it *is* important that the risks associated with vaccination are discussed and understood, there is a need to *balance* this information with the many positive benefits of immunisation.

Dangerous devices

One other area of concern is the relative ease by which patients can buy DIY health devices on the Internet. As long ago as 1997 the US Food and Drug Administration published a warning to consumers that home abortion kits posed 'significant, possibly life threatening health risks'. A subsequent health hazard assessment concluded that the use of this kit without a physician's supervision could 'cause heavy vaginal bleeding and even death'.

The sale of genetic testing kits over the Internet is another concern. Leaving aside the fact that the sale of such tests is unregulated (anyone can offer this service and provide all sorts of misleading and inaccurate information to patients), is it debateable whether these tests should be sold directly to patients, where the results will be read and acted upon without any input from a health professional.

HIV home testing kits are also readily available over the Internet. According to Professor Jonathon Weeber (an expert in HIV) home tests such as these are not as accurate as laboratory-based tests <http://news.bbc.co.uk/1/hi/health/1144066.stm> and consequently there is a risk that some people with HIV will delay seeking appropriate care, believing that the results of their home test were accurate.

Quality initiatives

In an attempt to protect consumers from the types of information (and products) discussed here, a number of organisations have developed mechanisms to evaluate Web sites and give 'badges of approval' to those that meet a defined quality threshold.

One of the more successful schemes has been developed by the Geneva-based Health on the Net Foundation (HON). Here, Web sites that comply with an eight-point Code of Conduct are granted the right to display the Health on the Net logo on their pages (**Figure 9.1**).

Central to this Code is the principle that any medical information must 'only be given by medically trained and qualified professionals'. Where this condition cannot be met there must be a 'clear statement that a piece of advice offered is from a non-medically qualified individual or organisation'. Full details of the Code can be found at: <http://www.hon.ch/HONcode/Conduct.html>.

The American Accreditation Healthcare Commission (URAC) has also developed a badging system to validate medical Web sites <http://webapps.urac.org/websiteaccreditation/Portal/Consumer/Index.asp>. Web sites that receive the URAC Health Web Site Accreditation Seal have

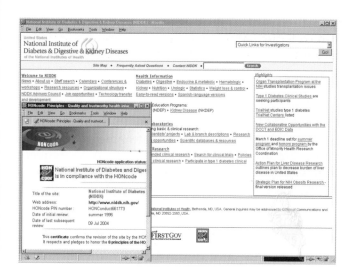

Figure 9.1   *The National Institute of Diabetes and Digestive and Kidney Diseases of the National and the Health on the Net logo – a sign of quality*

been evaluated against more than 50 Web site standards, covering topics such as quality of information, respect of privacy and issues relating to disclosure, and conflicts of interest.

Undoubtedly, the development of these badging systems is of benefit to the health information seeker. If you happen to come across a site that displays one of these badges you can be assured that the information will be of a high quality.

However, we do not believe that systems will ever provide all the solutions to the quality issue. There are simply too many health sites to badge – and if we took the simplistic view that you should only use those sites that have been badged you will exclude the majority of health Web sites. To put this in context, sites such as the National Cancer Institute, NHSDirect or the *BMJ* – all of which provide high-quality information – would have to be ignored as none of these display any 'quality assured' badge.

A more realistic solution is to encourage all Internet users to critically appraise and evaluate the information they find on the Internet.

Evaluating medical information

Critical appraisal is something most of us do all the time, albeit subconsciously. Thus, a news item broadcast by the BBC will tend to be believed, whereas a story in a tabloid newspaper may be treated with more caution.

On the Internet, however, where many of the sites are new and have not yet been able to build up a reputation for providing quality information, the appraisal process is more difficult, especially as sites of widely differing quality and with very different objectives may have confusingly similar Web addresses.

One simple way to evaluate information on the Internet is to use the four-point checklist, developed by Silberg and the American Medical Association (**Box 9.2**). Sites that fail to comply with these minimum standards should be rejected.

Box 9.2   Evaluating Web pages – Silberg criteria

♦ **Authorship**

The author(s) of a Web page, along with their affiliations and credentials should be clearly stated.

♦ **Attribution**

If a Web site is citing research or evidence then the source of this data must be explicitly stated. Ideally, there should be a hypertext link to the original research.

♦ **Disclosure**

The owner of the Web site must be prominently displayed, along with any sponsorship or advertising deals that could constitute a potential conflict of interest.

♦ **Currency**

Web pages should indicate when they were first created and last updated.

Based on the recommendations developed by Silberg WM, Lundberg GD, Musacchio RA. Assessing, controlling, and assuring the quality of medical information on the Internet: caveant lector et viewor – let the reader and viewer beware. *JAMA* 1997; **277**: 1244–5.

Top Tip

Nurses who are interested in developing their critical appraisal skills are encouraged to look at the DISCERN Instrument <http://www.discern.org.uk>. Based on 15 questions, this rating tool provides users with a 'valid and reliable way of assessing the quality of written information on treatment choices for a health problem'.

Conclusion

As anyone can set up a Web site and publish whatever they like, all Internet users need to be alert to the dangers of misleading, inaccurate and biased information.

However, using the tools, techniques and services discussed here, you can develop the necessary critical appraisal skills to assess what you find on the Internet. Armed with these skills – and those acquired during the course of this book – the true potential of the Internet can now be realised.

Glossary

Adobe Acrobat Reader
The Adobe Acrobat Reader is a piece of software – available free of charge – that can be used to read files created in a PDF format (see below).

Athens
Athens is an access management system that provides users with a single sign-on to numerous web-based services throughout the UK and overseas.

Binary files
A binary file is a file whose content must be interpreted by a computer program that understands in advance exactly how it is formatted. A document created in a word processor is an example of a binary file.

Boolean operators
The Boolean operators AND, OR, NOT (or AND NOT), and NEAR tell search engines which keywords you want your results to include or exclude, and whether you require that your keywords appear close to each other. The search 'cat AND dog' means find documents that mention cats and dogs, whilst the search 'cat OR dog' means find documents that discuss *either* concept.

Download
Downloading is the process of transferring (or copying) a file from a remote computer to your computer, usually over the Internet.

FAQ
Frequently asked questions.

Hypertext
Hypertext is text that contains links to other texts, pages and images.

MeSH subject headings
Developed by the US National Library of Medicine, 'Medical Subject Headings' is a controlled vocabulary and is used for indexing, cataloguing, and searching for biomedical and health-related information and documents.

Natural language searching
As the name implies, natural language searching allows the user to search for items using everyday, natural language. Natural

language searching is easier to use than controlled vocabularies (see MeSH) – but the search results may be less precise or comprehensive.

Newsgroup

An online, subject-specific, discussion group. There are many thousands of newsgroups on the Internet, covering every conceivable (and inconceivable!) subject.

PDF

Portable Document Format. To read a file created in this format you need software, such as the Adobe Acrobat Reader.

Peer-reviewed

Articles that have been peer-reviewed have been assessed to ensure that the research is scientifically sound. In essence it is a quality control and certification filter necessitated by the vast scale of learned research published today.

QuickTime

Developed by Apple, QuickTime is a piece of free software for listening to audio and watching video clips on the Internet.

Real Player

Developed by Real.com, Real Player is a piece of free software for listening to audio and watching video clips on the Internet.

Server

A server is a computer that provides services or resources to other computers.

Spam

Another term for junk (unwanted) electronic mail.

URL's

Uniform Resource Locators. The global address of documents and other resources on the Web.

Viruses

A computer program or piece of code that is loaded on to your computer without your knowledge and runs against your wishes.

Index

Page references to *figures, tables and boxes* are shown in *italics*